ON

ORTHOPAEDICS

M000198411

ON CALL
ORTHOPAEDICS

DOUGLAS R. DIRSCHL, MD
Assistant Professor of Orthopaedics
University of North Carolina School of Medicine
Wake Medical Education Institute
Raleigh, North Carolina

C. MICHAEL LeCROY, MD
Assistant Professor of Orthopaedics
University of North Carolina School of Medicine
Wake Medical Education Institute
Raleigh, North Carolina

With Contributions by

WILLIAM T. OBREMSKEY, MD, MPH
Assistant Professor of Orthopaedics
University of North Carolina School of Medicine
Wake Medical Education Institute
Raleigh, North Carolina

W.B. SAUNDERS COMPANY
A Division of Harcourt Brace & Company
Philadelphia London Toronto Montreal Sydney Tokyo

W.B. SAUNDERS COMPANY

A Division of Harcourt Brace & Company

The Curtis Center
Independence Square West
Philadelphia, Pennsylvania 19106

Library of Congress Cataloging-in-Publication Data

Dirschl, Douglas R.
    On call orthopaedics / Douglas R. Dirschl, C. Michael LeCroy :
with contributions by William T. Obremskey. — 1st ed.
        p.   cm.
    Includes index.
    ISBN 0-7216-7990-0
    1. Orthopaedics—Handbooks, manuals, etc.   2. Pediatric
orthopaedics—Handbooks, manuals, etc.   3. Musculoskeletal
emergencies—Handbooks, manuals, etc.   I. LeCroy, C. Michael.
II. Obremskey, William T.   III. Title.
    [DNLM: 1. Orthopaedic handbooks.   WE 39 D611o 1998]
RD732.5.D56   1998
616.7—dc21
DNLM/DLC

                                                                98-3606

ON CALL ORTHOPAEDICS   ISBN 0-7216-7990-0

Copyright © 1998 by W.B. Saunders Company

All rights reserved. No part of this publication may be reproduced or transmitted in any form or by any means, electronic or mechanical, including
photocopy, recording, or any information storage and retrieval system,
without permission in writing from the publisher.

Printed in the United States of America

Last digit is the print number: 9   8   7   6   5   4   3   2   1

PREFACE

In teaching hospitals, calls from patient care units traditionally are directed to medical students and residents. In a discipline such as internal medicine, most calls originate from inpatient nursing units. In orthopaedics, however, calls originate from the emergency department at least as often as from inpatient nursing units. The orthopaedic consultant is thus confronted with calls from a variety of individuals who will present a variable amount of information at the time of consultation. It is our belief that preparation of the student or physician to undertake the duties of the orthopaedic consultant need not be a trial-and-error experience filled with anxiety and uncertainty.

On Call Orthopaedics takes as its mission the introduction of the medical student or resident to the assessment and management of musculoskeletal problems commonly encountered in hospital practice. It is not the purpose of this text to provide a complete, in-depth orthopaedic education—such an undertaking being the purview of standard, multiple-volume textbooks of orthopaedics. Rather, it is our intent that *On Call Orthopaedics* be an introductory text, pocket guide, and reference source for the student or physician called to evaluate and manage patients with acute or chronic musculoskeletal disorders. Although problems such as abdominal pain, dysuria, and shortness of breath can occur in all hospitalized patients, orthopaedic or otherwise, this text addresses only musculoskeletal complaints. The authors refer the reader to other sources for information about the management of nonmusculoskeletal disorders.

Problem-oriented medical education has taken root throughout North America, and this text attempts, wherever possible, to adopt a similar approach. After an introductory section on general terminology and principles, the remainder of the text is devoted to common musculoskeletal complaints for which a resident or medical student is likely to be called. The text is further divided into musculoskeletal complaints in the absence of traumatic injury, complaints following traumatic injury, and conditions specific to children. As with the entire *On Call* series, this text contains a formulary of frequently prescribed medications for patients with musculoskeletal problems. It is our hope the reader will find *On Call Orthopaedics* a valuable reference source for the evaluation and management of patients with musculoskeletal complaints.

Douglas R. Dirschl
C. Michael LeCroy

COMMONLY USED ABBREVIATIONS

AC	acromioclavicular joint
ACL	anterior cruciate ligament
ADL	activities of daily living
AP	anteroposterior
AS	ankylosing spondylitis
ATLS	advanced trauma life support
AVN	avascular necrosis
B	bilateral
CBC	complete blood count
CRP	C-reactive protein
CT	computed tomography
CTS	carpal tunnel syndrome
DDD	degenerative disk disease
DDH	developmental dysplasia of the hip
DIP	distal interphalangeal
DJD	degenerative joint disease
DM	diabetes mellitus
DVT	deep vein thrombosis
ESR	erythrocyte sedimentation rate
F/E	flexion/extension
FX	fracture
HIV	human immunodeficiency virus
HNP	herniated nucleus pulposus
HV	hallux valgus
IM	intramuscular, intramedullary
IV	intravenous
JRA	juvenile rheumatoid arthritis
L	left

LAC	long arm cast
LAT	lateral
LBP	low back pain
LCL	lateral collateral ligament
LCP	Legg-Calvé-Perthes disease
LLC	long leg cast
LR	lactated Ringer's solution
MAST	military antishock trousers
MCL	medial collateral ligament
MCP	metacarpophalangeal
MRI	magnetic resonance imaging
MSK	musculoskeletal
MTP	metatarsophalangeal
MVA	motor vehicle accident
MVC	motor vehicle crash
NS	normal saline
NSAIDs	nonsteroidal anti-inflammatory drugs
NV	neurovascular
OA	osteoarthritis
OCD	osteochondritis dissecans
OR	operating room
PCL	posterior cruciate ligament
PIP	proximal interphalangeal
PT	physical therapy
R	right
RA	rheumatoid arthritis
RN	registered nurse
ROM	range of motion
SAC	short arm cast
SCD	sickle cell disease
SCFE	slipped capital femoral epiphysis
SLC	short leg cast

SLR	straight leg raise
STS	sugar tong splint
TEV	talipes equinovarus
US	ultrasound
V/V	varus/valgus
VS	vital signs
WB	weight bearing
WBAT	weight bearing as tolerated
WBC	white blood cell
XR	x-ray, radiograph

CONTENTS

GENERAL INFORMATION

PATIENT-RELATED PROBLEMS
Problems Without Associated Trauma
(Overuse and Degenerative Conditions)

Problems with Associated Trauma

PROBLEMS PARTICULAR TO CHILDREN

APPENDIXES

GENERAL INFORMATION

ORTHOPAEDIC TERMINOLOGY

Douglas R. Dirschl

To fully understand the pathologic conditions of the musculoskeletal system and to be able to easily communicate musculoskeletal findings to others, it is necessary to understand and be able to correctly use several important clinical terms in the musculoskeletal language. Many of the terms listed below are pairs that have opposite meanings and, as such, can frequently be confused by medical students and young physicians. The terms listed below describe movements of joints, deformities of limbs, and orthopaedic procedures and therefore are used frequently in discussions of musculoskeletal conditions. Once the student or resident has learned these terms thoroughly, they will become mainstays of the musculoskeletal vocabulary.

■ TERMS DESCRIBING MOVEMENTS OF JOINTS

Active movement: Movement of a joint that occurs as a result of the power of the individual's own muscular activity. For example, active movement of the knee can be tested by asking the seated patient to extend and flex the knee.

Passive movement: Movement of a joint that occurs as the result of an external force, usually the force of an examining physician. For example, passive movement of the knee can be tested by having the relaxed patient allow the knee to be flexed and extended by the examining physician.

Abduction: The movement of a body part away from the midline. Abduction occurs primarily at the hip and shoulder joints.

Adduction: The movement of a body part toward the midline. Adduction also occurs primarily at the hip and shoulder joints.

Dorsiflexion: The movement of the ankle or toes in the direction of the dorsal surface. It also refers to movement of the wrist or fingers in the direction of the dorsal surface.

Plantar flexion: The movement of the ankle or toes in the direction of the plantar surface.

Palmar flexion: The movement of the wrist or fingers in the direction of the palmar surface.

Eversion: The turning of the plantar surface of the foot outward in relation to the leg.

Inversion: The turning of the plantar surface of the foot inward in relation to the leg. Most ankle sprains occur with the foot in inversion.

Internal rotation: The turning of the anterior surface of the limb inward or medially. An example of internal rotation of the hips involves standing pigeon-toed.

External rotation: The turning of the anterior surface of the limb outward or laterally. An example of external rotation of the hips involves standing with the toes pointing outward.

Pronation of the forearm: The turning of the palmar surface of the hand downward or toward the posterior surface of the body.

Supination of the forearm: The turning of the palmar surface of the hand upward or toward the anterior surface of the body.

■ TERMS DESCRIBING DEFORMITIES IN LIMBS

Static deformities: Rigid deformities, resistant to passive correction, that remain the same regardless of the position in which the limb is placed.

Flexible deformities: Deformities that generally are not resistant to passive correction (are mobile) and that occur as a result of the patient's own muscle action.

Calcaneus deformity: A deformity in which the ankle is maintained in a position of dorsiflexion so that, on weightbearing, only the heel touches the floor. (Do not confuse with the largest bone in the foot, also called the calcaneus.)

Equinus deformity: A deformity in which the ankle is maintained in a position of plantar flexion so that, on weightbearing, only the forefoot and toes touch the floor.

Pes: Foot

Pes cavus: An exaggeration of the normal longitudinal arch of the foot, creating an unusually high arch.

Pes planus: A flattening of the normal longitudinal arc of the foot, an unduly low arch or flatfoot.

Varus deformity: An abnormal angulation of the limb in which the distal portion is directed toward the midline of the body.

    Cubitus varus: A decrease in the normal carrying angle at the elbow (also known as the "gunstock deformity").

    Coxa vara: A decrease in the femoral neck–shaft angle at the hip.

    Genu varum: Bowleg(s), the knees are apart when the feet are together.

    Talipes equinovarus: Commonly known as clubfoot. This is an inversion deformity of the forefoot combined with equinus deformity of the ankle.

Valgus deformity: An abnormal angulation of the limb in which the distal portion is directed away from the midline of the body.

Cubitus valgus: An increase in the normal carrying angle at the elbow.

Coxa valga: An increase in the femoral neck–shaft angle at the hip.

Genu valgum: Knock knee(s), the feet are apart when the knees are together.

Talipes calcaneovalgus: An eversion deformity of the foot combined with dorsiflexion deformity of the ankle. Commonly seen in cerebral palsy and myelomeningocele.

Hallux valgus: An abduction deformity of the great toe through the metatarsophalangeal joint (also known as bunion).

■ TERMS DESCRIBING OPERATIVE PROCEDURES

Osteotomy: The cutting of a bone, usually to correct deformity.

Arthrodesis: The operative fusion of a joint.

Arthroplasty: The operative reconstruction of a joint to restore motion and relieve pain. Arthroplasty may or may not include the implantation of synthetic joint components, as in a total hip arthroplasty.

Osteosynthesis: The procedure for reconstructing bones that have been fractured. Osteosynthesis can be accomplished by various means, including screws, plates and screws, intramedullary devices, and external skeletal fixators.

■ TERMS DESCRIBING PARTS OF A LONG BONE (Fig. 1–1)

Diaphysis: The shaft of a long bone. The diaphysis is the strong, tubular portion of the bone that comprises, in most long bones, the majority of its length.

Metaphysis: The spongy part of a long bone that extends from the diaphysis to the articular surface at the end of a long bone.

Epiphysis: The very end segment of a long bone, which was formed by a secondary center of ossification and supports the overlying articular cartilage.

Physis: Also known as the growth plate, the physis is the area of the long bone from which longitudinal growth occurs. The physis generally closes in most long bones in the teenage years, at which time, longitudinal skeletal growth ceases.

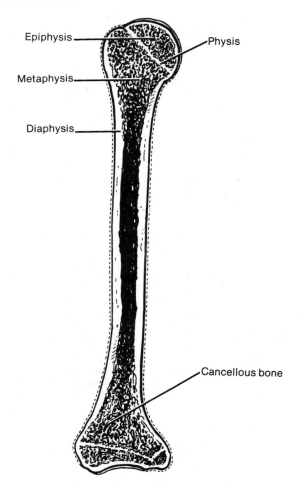

Figure 1–1 □ Parts of a long bone. (From Gartland JJ. Fundamentals of Orthopaedics, 4th ed. Philadelphia, WB Saunders, 1986.)

Apophysis: A secondary growth center within bone that grows under tension, usually by the pull of a muscle or tendon. The most commonly encountered apophyses are at the greater trochanter of the femur, the tibial tubercle of the proximal tibia, the insertion of the Achilles tendon on the calcaneus, and the medial epicondyle at the elbow. Apophyses generally remain open longer than do physes, and some apophyses may not close until late in the third decade of life.

2

ORDERING AND INTERPRETING MUSCULOSKELETAL RADIOGRAPHS

Douglas R. Dirschl

The diagnostic evaluation of the orthopaedic patient is a puzzle often easily solved. The history and physical examination are the most important means of evaluating the patient with musculoskeletal complaints, and on many occasions no additional diagnostic information is necessary. In other instances, however, diagnostic evaluation requires integration of information from additional sources, and diagnostic imaging most frequently provides the necessary additional information.

The most common diagnostic imaging modality for the orthopaedic patient is conventional radiography (x-ray), which is the cornerstone of imaging the musculoskeletal system. Radiographic facilities to perform these studies are relatively inexpensive and are located in nearly all clinical settings. High quality radiography, however, requires carefully calibrated and maintained equipment, proper processing, and well-trained technical personnel. Appropriately trained personnel are particularly important, since proper selection of radiographic technique and accurate positioning are vital for optimal results with conventional radiography.

Conventional radiographs are obtained in nearly all patients with musculoskeletal complaints. Although a large proportion of patients with musculoskeletal complaints have no bony pathology, radiographs are nonetheless important to exclude other, more severe conditions that may involve the bone (e.g., chronic infection, stress fracture, malignancy). Ordering the correct radiographs for a given musculoskeletal complaint requires some foreknowledge and experience. For a listing of the appropriate radiographs to order for a variety of musculoskeletal complaints, please see the relevant chapters in Section II: Patient Related Problems: the Common Calls. This chapter is devoted to some basic principles to be followed in ordering and interpreting musculoskeletal radiographs.

■ ORDERING ORTHOPAEDIC RADIOGRAPHS

1. When obtaining radiographs of the musculoskeletal system, the physician should order at least two orthogonal radiographic views. Most commonly, these views will be an anteroposterior (AP) view and a lateral view of the area to be

imaged. Dislocations and fractures may be apparent on only one of the two orthogonal views. Always ordering at least two orthogonal views of the area of concern will keep the physician from falling prey to the old orthopaedic adage that "one view is no view."

2. Particularly when imaging a suspected fracture in a long bone, it is advisable to order radiographs that include at least one joint above and one joint below the area of concern. Fractures can extend from the diaphysis (shaft) of a bone to the articular surface, and particularly in the forearm and leg, fractures of one bone can be associated with dislocations of the joints at either end. For example, a fracture of the ulnar shaft may be associated with a dislocation of the radial head at the elbow. This is termed a *Monteggia fracture* and can easily be missed if radiographs do not include the elbow joint.

3. Most hospital radiology departments have simplified the process of ordering radiographs by grouping the most common and most useful radiographic views of a given region into a series. An example of this is a knee series, which generally includes AP, lateral, intercondylar notch, and sunrise views. If, when ordering musculoskeletal radiographs, the physician is in doubt about what views would be the most useful, a good rule of thumb is to order a series. For example, ordering an ankle series obtains three useful views of the ankle—AP, lateral, and mortise views.

4. When ordering musculoskeletal radiographs of regions that are painful only with use (especially in the lower limb), the physician should consider obtaining radiographs of those regions when they are in use. For example, a patient with knee pain that occurs only with standing and walking should have radiographs of the knee made while standing. If this patient has degenerative arthritis, the standing radiograph may show narrowing of the medial joint space and varus deformity of the knee, whereas a non-weight-bearing radiograph might show a normal joint space and normal alignment. Another example is the patient with a painful flatfoot; radiographs of the foot with the patient bearing weight are much more useful to the clinician than non-weight-bearing radiographs are.

■ INTERPRETATION OF MUSCULOSKELETAL RADIOGRAPHS

Many students, resident physicians, and nonmusculoskeletal specialists have difficulty interpreting musculoskeletal radiographs. This difficulty usually stems from inexperience and a lack of comfort viewing bone radiographs, rather than from any inherent complexity in the radiographs themselves. Although a resident or medical student cannot expect to interpret all musculoskeletal radiographs with the ease and accuracy of an orthopaedist or a radiologist, some general rules are helpful in identifying abnormalities on musculoskeletal radiographs:

1. When viewing musculoskeletal radiographs, always determine first what area has been imaged and what views have been obtained. For example, beginning the interpretation of radiographs of the hand by understanding that AP, lateral, and oblique views of the hand were obtained is of great help in understanding the anatomic relationships of the bones and any abnormalities that may be encountered.

2. Be certain to identify all the bony structures on the radiograph, correctly naming each bone as you do. This not only is an excellent exercise in reviewing the bony anatomy of that particular region but also is necessary if one is to accurately describe the radiographic findings to another physician. It is embarrassing to describe over the telephone a fracture of the radius, only to be corrected later by the orthopaedist, who informs you the fracture is in the ulna rather than the radius.

3. It is important to remember that although a musculoskeletal radiograph is a diagnostic image, it can often be accurately interpreted only by correlation with the patient's symptoms and the clinical examination. For example, a patient with lateral ankle pain and tenderness but no medial tenderness requires careful assessment of the distal fibula on radiographs, with less attention being paid to the medial malleolus. The physician must keep in mind that old skeletal injuries may appear as abnormalities on skeletal radiographs but are not necessarily the cause of the patient's current symptoms. In the above example of the patient with lateral ankle pain the presence of an old, healed fracture of the medial malleolus is an abnormal radiographic finding but is not at all associated with the patient's present complaint of lateral ankle pain.

4. The cortical outline of every *normal* bone on a radiograph will consist of smooth contours and corners. At no time is it normal for a bone to have a sudden step-off or sharp angulation of the cortical margin. Carefully outlining the cortical margins of the bone of interest can be helpful in identifying subtle fractures not readily apparent on initial perusal of the radiograph (Fig. 2–1A).

5. In interpreting radiographs in skeletally immature individuals, it is important to remember that many physes (growth plates) do not close until the late teenage years. Physes almost always run transversely at the ends of long bones and can easily be mistaken for fractures (Fig. 2–1B). It is extremely important to correlate the clinical findings with the radiographic findings in the area of a growth plate. A growth plate that is not tender on physical examination is rarely abnormal on radiographs. A growth plate that is tender on clinical examina-

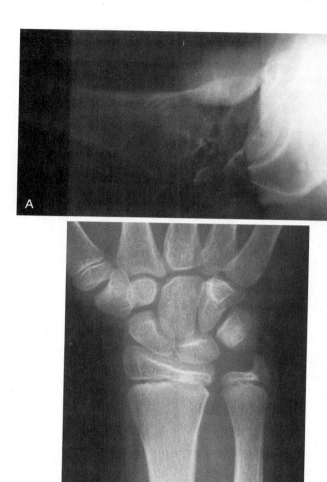

Figure 2–1 □ **A,** Lateral radiograph of a hip showing a fracture of the femoral neck. The posterior cortex of the femoral neck is seen to have a sharp angulation at the fracture site. **B,** AP radiograph of a normal wrist in a growing child. The transverse radiolucent lines in the distal radius and ulna are growth plates, rather than fractures.

tion, however, may have an occult fracture, even though radiographs fail to demonstrate any abnormality.

■ DESCRIPTION OF FRACTURES AND DISLOCATIONS

Fractures of bones and dislocations of joints are commonly seen on radiographs following musculoskeletal injury. It can be exceedingly difficult, however, for the physician to accurately describe the fracture pattern over the telephone. Keeping a few simple terms in mind can simplify the task of describing radiographs of fractures or dislocations.

A fracture can occur in any region within a bone and may be entirely outside of a joint (extraarticular) or may extend into a joint (intraarticular). There are also various named regions within the extraarticular portions of long bones (see Fig. 1–1). The *metaphysis* lies between the *physis* (growth plate) and the long tubular portion

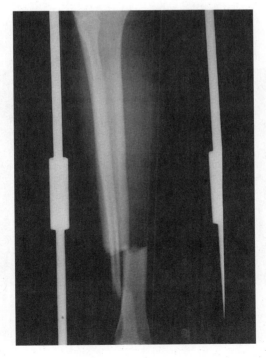

Figure 2–2 □ Transverse fractures of the shafts of the tibia and fibula.

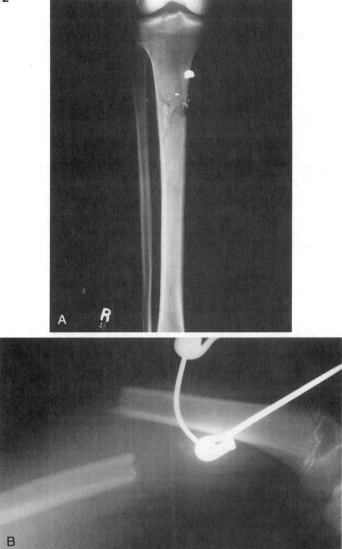

Figure 2–3 □ **A,** Nondisplaced fracture of the proximal tibia caused by a gunshot wound. Note that although there is fracture comminution, the overall alignment of the bone remains anatomic. **B,** A lateral radiograph of a fracture of the distal femur in which the distal fragment is displaced anteriorly relative to the proximal fragment. This is referred to as *anterior displacement.* There is a traction pin in the distal fragment.

of the bone, which is termed the *diaphysis*. The *epiphysis* is the portion of the bone between the physis and the articular surface; hence, the epiphysis is always intraarticular.

Once the location of the fracture has been identified, the physician should identify the fracture pattern. A *transverse fracture* extends directly across a long bone, perpendicular to the long axis of the bone (Fig. 2–2). An *oblique fracture* is at an angle to the long axis of the bone such that the two ends may slide relative to one another. A *spiral fracture* occurs as a result of a twisting injury and is characterized by a spiraling pattern of the fracture, such that one cannot see clearly through the fracture on either the AP or lateral radiographic views. A *comminuted fracture* is one in which there are numerous free fragments attached to neither the main proximal nor distal part of the fractured bone.

Once the location and pattern of the fracture have been determined, the next step is to determine the relationship between the

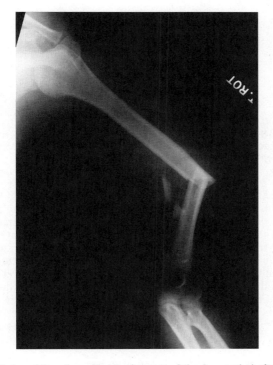

Figure 2–4 □ AP radiograph of a fracture of the humeral shaft in which both fractured bone ends point toward the lateral (radial) side of the arm. The fracture is said to have apex lateral (radial) angulation.

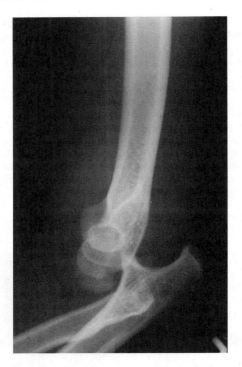

Figure 2–5 □ A lateral radiograph of an elbow dislocation in which the ulna is displaced posterior to the distal humerus. This is referred to as a *posterior dislocation* of the elbow.

two major fracture fragments. A fracture is *nondisplaced* if the two major fracture fragments have complete contact with one another on both the AP and lateral radiographs (Fig. 2–3*A*). A fracture is *partially displaced* if there is at least some contact between the two fracture fragments on AP and lateral radiographs. A fracture is *completely displaced* if there is no contact between the fracture fragments on the AP or lateral radiographs. The direction of displacement of the fracture is described as the relationship of the distal fragment to the proximal fragment. For example, a patient with a transverse fracture of the femoral shaft in which the distal fragment of the fracture is displaced anteriorly relative to the proximal fragment is described as an *anteriorly displaced fracture of the femoral shaft* (Fig. 2–3*B*).

Angulation of a fracture is present when the two fracture fragments do not form a straight line along the normal axis of the long bone. Angulation is described by the direction in which the apex of the angular deformity points. For example, a humeral shaft fracture in which the two fragments both point toward the lateral (radial) surface of the arm is said to have apex lateral (radial) angulation (Fig. 2–4). The magnitude of the angulation is determined by direct measurement on the radiographs using a goniometer.

Displacement is defined similarly for *dislocated joints*, where again the relationship of the distal bone to the proximal bone is used to describe the direction of dislocation. For example, a dislocation of the elbow joint in which the ulna and radius are displaced posterior to the distal humerus is termed a *posterior dislocation of the elbow* (Fig. 2–5).

In summary, when describing fractures of the long bones, first name the bone and identify the location of the fracture in the bone, then identify the fracture pattern, then identify the direction and magnitude of any displacement or angulation of the fractured bone ends. For dislocations of joints, first identify the name of the joint, then identify the relationship between the distal and proximal bones to describe the direction of dislocation of the joint.

Adherence to some basic principles in the ordering, interpretation, and description of musculoskeletal radiographs can demystify these tests, which are sometimes felt to be difficult to perform and accurately interpret. Experience, combined with adherence to some simple principles and techniques, can make the evaluation and description of musculoskeletal radiographs much easier.

3

PRINCIPLES OF ORTHOPAEDIC CARE

Douglas R. Dirschl

In clinical practice, patients present with a wide variety of disorders and injuries to the musculoskeletal system. In addition, the same disorder or injury may present different problems for different patients. For example, a fractured great toe may be much more disabling for a ballet dancer than for a taxi driver. It is not surprising, therefore, that the methods of treatment for patients with musculoskeletal disorders are both numerous and varied. It is unnecessary for the physician to know every possible method of treatment for a given musculoskeletal condition. If the physician has an understanding of the goals and principles underlying the treatment of musculoskeletal conditions, most of the specific treatment methods will become evident. The purpose of this chapter is to give a brief synopsis of the goals and principles for treating musculoskeletal conditions.

■ TREATMENT GOALS

The major goals of treating musculoskeletal conditions are surprisingly simple:
1. Decrease pain
2. Avoid morbidity
3. Promote the return of normal functioning

Patients with musculoskeletal injuries or disorders frequently have a great deal of pain. The function of the musculoskeletal system is to allow the human body to move fluidly; attempts at movement or resumption of regular activities in the presence of a musculoskeletal disorder or injury can result in great pain. Therefore one of the earliest and primary goals in treating musculoskeletal conditions is to relieve pain.

As a result of many important advances in the field of medicine, physicians have at their disposal a plethora of powerful and effective methods of treating patients with musculoskeletal problems. The physician must keep in mind that although these methods have potential for great benefit, they also have the potential to cause great harm. The Hippocratic dictum *"first do no harm"* is applicable to all areas of medicine. The physician must be constantly aware of the potential complications of treatment and plan his or her treatment to give the greatest benefit to the patient while minimizing the potential for morbidity.

The physician treating the patient with a musculoskeletal injury or disorder must also keep in mind that he or she must not simply treat bones and joints but rather must treat the *patient*. For example, since the function of the musculoskeletal system is to allow movement and strength, a united fracture or a healed ligament is of little benefit to the patient if the limb cannot function normally. Thus, promoting a return to normal functioning is one of the primary goals of treatment of musculoskeletal conditions.

The treatment goals listed above can be summed up in a statement by Sir Robert Jones, an English orthopaedist of the 19th and early 20th centuries, who said "the object of treatment is the restoration of complete function with the least risk and inconvenience to the patient."

■ TREATMENT METHODS

The treatment methods used for musculoskeletal disorders falls into three broad categories
1. No active treatment (i.e., reassurance alone)
2. Nonoperative treatment
3. Operative treatment

For every patient presenting with a musculoskeletal disorder, each of these three treatment possibilities should be considered, because the risk of complications increases with the aggressiveness of treatment. Approximately one half of patients with musculoskeletal complaints (excluding cases of fracture) attending outpatient clinics do not require active treatment. All that these patients need is reassurance, counseling, and education. In many cases the sole reason for the patient's attendance in the office or emergency department is that he or she fears having cancer, tuberculosis, impending paralysis, or some other serious condition. If patients can be reassured that there is no evidence of serious disease and that pain and disability are self-limiting, they will return home satisfied, and their symptoms may become less disturbing.

If active treatment seems to be required, it is a good general principle that, whenever practical, treatment should begin with a trial of nonoperative measures. The physician should keep in mind that most orthopaedic surgical procedures are "semielective," rather than emergency, lifesaving procedures. Consequently the patient with a degenerative or overuse disorder should seldom be persuaded to submit immediately to operation. Instead, the patient, after an unsuccessful trial of nonoperative treatment, should persuade the surgeon to undertake surgery. If the physician is undecided whether to advise nonoperative or operative treatment, it is generally wise to err on the side of nonoperative treatment. This book does not discuss the operative treatment of musculoskeletal injuries and disorders.

■ NONOPERATIVE TREATMENT

Rest

In the nineteenth century the English bone setter Hugh Owen Thomas emphasized the value of rest in diseases of the spine and limbs. Since that time, rest has been one of the mainstays of musculoskeletal treatment. While complete rest was sometimes advocated in the past, the current preference is for *relative rest,* a term that implies a reduction in overall activity and particularly in activities that cause pain in the injured part. For example, for a distance runner who experiences heel pain after running 6 miles, relative rest might involve running shorter distances or performing cross-training activities, such as cycling or swimming. Similarly, for acute low back pain, prolonged bed rest is no longer recommended. Instead, 24 to 48 hours of complete rest is recommended, followed by gradually increasing activity, while avoiding stooping, lifting, or other activities that increase strain on the lumbar spine.

Support

Rest and support generally complement one another, but there are occasions where support is desired but rest is not. For example, after repair of fractured metacarpals in the hand, support is needed to reduce pain and prevent reinjury, but immediate motion of the hand and fingers is also needed to avoid stiffness of the fingers. When support is to be temporary, it can be provided by a splint, either a commercially available splint or one made of plaster of Paris or fiberglass. When support is to be prolonged, a custom-made orthosis or cast is required. When support is to be permanent, a custom-made appliance or orthosis generally is recommended.

Physiotherapy

Physiotherapy in its various forms occupies an important place in the nonoperative as well as in the postoperative treatment of musculoskeletal disorders. Since physiotherapy is easily prescribed and entails no additional effort on the part of the physician, it frequently is overused. A great deal of physiotherapy is prescribed that can have no physically beneficial effect for the patient. Judicious and appropriate use of physiotherapy can increase range of motion, decrease swelling and inflammation, and speed the recovery of function for patients with musculoskeletal injuries or disorders. It is important, however, to counsel patients that although physical therapy is an important part of treatment, a therapist will not make them better. A motivated, hard-working patient is a prerequisite to obtaining the maximum benefit of physiotherapy. A patient who makes half-hearted attempts at physiotherapy or who does not perform home exercise programs during the intervals between therapy appointments will likely gain little or no benefit from the physician's having prescribed physiotherapy. All patients should be counseled that they must take an active role in the rehabilitation of their musculoskeletal condition for the optimal return of function.

Local Injections

Local injections, either of anesthetics, corticosteroids, or a combination of the two, are used *infrequently* in the management of musculoskeletal conditions. The indications for local injections include the following:

1. Osteoarthritis or rheumatoid arthritis in which the medication, generally a corticosteroid, is injected directly into the affected joint with the goal of relieving inflammation and pain.
2. Extraarticular lesions of the type often described as a chronic strain. Examples include tennis elbow, tendinitis about the shoulder, and certain types of back pain.

The results following injection are technique dependent, and repeated injections in the same location can lead to tendon degeneration and perhaps rupture. Repeated intraarticular injections of corticosteroids are believed to accelerate the progression of osteoarthritis.

Pharmacotherapy

Pharmacotherapy has a rather small place in the practice of musculoskeletal medicine. Pharmacologic agents used for musculoskeletal disorders may be placed into six general categories: (1) antibacterial agents, (2) analgesics, (3) sedatives, (4) anti-inflammatory medications, and (5) hormonelike drugs.

Antibacterial agents are of immense importance in the treatment of infective lesions, particularly in acute osteomyelitis and acute pyogenic arthritis. To be successful, treatment must begin early in the disease course and must deliver the appropriate antibiotic to the infected site in an adequate concentration for a long enough time to eradicate the infection. Parenteral and oral antibiotic agents frequently are employed.

Analgesics should be used as infrequently as possible. While narcotic analgesic medications are effective at relieving acute pain, they have been proven relatively ineffective at relieving chronic pain. Many orthopaedic disorders are characterized by pain that may not resolve for weeks or months, and it is undesirable to prescribe any narcotic analgesic continually over long periods, except perhaps in the case of incurable malignant disease.

Anti-inflammatory agents decrease the inflammatory response that occurs following either acute or long-term injury. It is important to remember that inflammation is a normal but poorly understood response of the human body to injury. Although anti-inflammatory medications can decrease pain and inflammation, it is not absolutely known whether these medications actually speed healing and return to function following musculoskeletal injury. The most powerful anti-inflammatory medications are the corticosteroids. These agents should be used with extreme caution, because their side effects (such as avascular necrosis of the femoral head) can be serious. Nonsteroidal anti-inflammatory medications (NSAIDs), of which there are numerous types, generally are preferred, and they are a mainstay of the treatment of arthritic and degenerative conditions. Well-known examples are aspirin, indomethacin, and ibuprofen. Most of these medications also have an analgesic action and well-described side effects, particularly irritation to the lining of the gastrointestinal system. It is important to understand that the anti-inflammatory effect of the NSAIDs only occurs when the medication has reached a steady state serum level, whereas the analgesic effect of the medication occurs after each dose. Therefore a patient would need to take 3 to 5 days of a tid NSAID (i.e., ibuprofen) before a significant anti-inflammatory effect would be noted.

Hormonelike drugs include the corticosteroids noted above, as well as estrogen and its analogs, which are used for slowing the rate of bone mineral loss in early postmenopausal women who are at high risk for osteoporosis. Perhaps also to be included in this group of medications are the bisphosphonates, which, although relatively new, are gaining widespread use in decreasing the rate of bone loss in elderly patients with osteoporosis.

With an understanding of the principal goals of treating musculoskeletal conditions—decreasing pain, promoting return to function, and minimizing morbidity—the physician has a starting point from which to formulate individual treatment plans. With a further understanding of the general principles of nonoperative treatment of musculoskeletal conditions, the physician, even without an extensive knowledge of specific modes of therapy, can have a sufficient understanding to devise therapeutic methodologies that can be helpful to these patients.

4

PRINCIPLES OF SPLINTING

Douglas R. Dirschl

One of the most often touted and least frequently obeyed maxims in emergency care is "splint them where they lie." Even after examination by a physician in the emergency department, most patients are shuffled off for x-ray examination without having their injured limbs splinted. In addition, many patients arriving in the emergency department with splints in place have them removed before they are sent for radiographs. In one informal survey of five emergency departments, less than 20% of patients with fractures had their fractured limbs splinted before being seen by an orthopaedist.

Adequate and timely splinting is desirable for the following reasons:

1. Immobilization of fractured bones and injured soft tissues relieves pain.
2. Additional soft tissue injury (especially to nerves and blood vessels) may be prevented.
3. Splinting of closed fractures prevents them from becoming open fractures.
4. Splinting of long bone fractures may decrease hemorrhage and lower the incidence of fat embolism syndrome.
5. Splinting makes transporting the patient and obtaining radiographs easier for emergency department staff and less painful for the patient.

That no splints are available should never be used as an excuse for not splinting a fractured limb. Almost anything rigid can be pressed into service—crutches or canes, umbrellas, pieces of wood—padded by almost any soft material. When all else fails, bandaging the lower extremities together or fixing the arm to the trunk will help. For injuries of the ankle or foot, a pillow pinned or bandaged around the injured area immobilizes by its bulk.

Many hospital emergency departments stock a wide variety of prefabricated splints, usually made of metal with or without a vinyl coating, for the wrist, foot, and leg. While these splints are useful in selected circumstances for short durations (less than 2 hours), the most comfortable and most effective splints are those custom molded from plaster of Paris. Plaster of Paris splints should consist of at least ten layers of plaster casting material (at least five thicknesses of cast padding on each side of the splint) and an elastic bandage to hold the splint on the limb. A number of commercial products incorporate the plaster casting material and the padding (usually foam rubber) into a single unit; in our experience, splints made of these materials are less effective in stabilizing fractures, are far less comfortable for the patient, and result more frequently in pressure sores of the skin than do plaster splints made by the physician.

The *steps in making and applying a plaster splint* are as follows:

1. Cast padding should be used to measure for the length of splint necessary. Four to six inches (10 to 15 cm) extra should be added to the length of the splint, as plaster of Paris will shrink somewhat as it dries. This length of cast padding is then torn off of the roll and used as a template.

2. Plaster casting material is then laid out to the preselected width and length for the splint. In general, 10 to 15 thicknesses of plaster are adequate for splinting applications. Please refer to Table 4–1 for the widths of plaster used for the most common splinting applications in adults.

3. A single layer of cast padding wide enough to cover all of the plaster is then applied on top. The purpose of this cast padding is to make the splint cleaner to handle and easier to remove. If cast padding is not placed on the outside of the splint, the elastic bandage will stick to the plaster, and the splint will be difficult to remove.

4. A minimum of five thicknesses of cast padding are then applied to the other side of the splint. Fewer than five thicknesses does not adequately pad the patient's skin, and pain or skin breakdown may occur in areas of increased pressure.

5. The plaster is then wet, and excess water is squeezed from the splint. The layers of the splint are then laminated together by rubbing them with the hands.

6. The splint is then assembled with the wet plaster splinting material sandwiched between the dry layers of cast padding.

7. The assembled wet splint is then applied to the limb with the limb held in the desired position.

8. Elastic bandages are then used to wrap the splint to the limb. It is important that the elastic bandages secure the splint firmly to the limb; however, the elastic bandages should not be so tight as to restrict the circulation to the limb. As a general rule, if one can easily insert a finger beneath the edge of an ap-

Table 4–1 □ **WIDTHS OF COMMON PLASTER OF PARIS SPLINTS**

Splint	Width of Plaster Required
Thumb spica	3 inches (7.5 cm)
Wrist (volar)	4 inches (10 cm)
Sugar tong (wrist and elbow)	4 inches (10 cm)
U splint (humerus)	4 inches (10 cm)
All lower limb splints	5 or 6 inches (12.5 or 15 cm)

plied elastic bandage, the bandage has not been wrapped too tightly.

9. The completed splint is then molded to the extremity and the extremity held securely in the desired position until the plaster has hardened. The large, meaty surfaces of the thenar and hypothenar eminences of the hands should be used to mold plaster; pressure should never be applied with the fingertips. The result of molding or pressing plaster with the fingertips will be a series of indentations on the outer surface of the finished splint, which may create pressure points against the patient's skin. It is also important to note that plaster is weakest just as it begins to set. This is a critical time, and the limb must be held still in the desired position until the plaster has completely hardened.

Specific Splints

As a general rule, splints should immobilize the joints above and below the site of suspected injury (e.g., immobilize the elbow and wrist if the forearm is injured). The following are *splinting techniques* for various areas:

Spine	Place the patient on a spine board with sandbags on each side of the head to prevent rotation of the neck.
Neck	Utilize a hard cervical collar or a spine board as above.
Shoulder	Use a sling and swathe for shoulder injuries unless a shoulder dislocation prevents positioning the arm across the chest.
Humerus	Use a U splint beginning in the axilla and extending around the elbow, up the arm, and ending above the shoulder. The arm should then also be supported in a sling and swathe.
Elbow and forearm	Use a posterior splint extending from just below the shoulder to the metacarpals.
Wrist and hand	Use a volar splint for wrist and hand injuries, extending from the palm to just below the elbow. If the patient has severe deformity from a distal radial fracture, one should consider a sugar tong splint, which extends from the palm, up the volar forearm, around the elbow, and down the dorsal forearm to end over the dorsum of the hand.
Hip and femur	Dislocations of the hip produce a flexion/adduction deformity that should not be corrected during splinting. If flexion deformity is present, use pillows or folded blankets to support the leg as it lies. Femur fractures can be splinted for several hours using a commercially available splint that applies skin traction.
Knee	Most knee injuries can be immobilized with well-padded, medial and lateral plaster splints from groin to ankle. Many knee injuries can also be immobilized with a simple, commercially available knee immobilizer.

Tibia	Splints for tibial fractures must control both the ankle and knee. Well-padded plaster slabs from groin to toes are generally recommended. Splints extending to just below the knee are not adequate to stabilize tibial shaft fractures.
Ankle	If a fracture of the ankle involves both malleoli, the splint must extend from the thigh to the toes. Otherwise, apply a plaster splint shaped into a U extending from the medial side of the leg around the heel and up the lateral side of the leg. Combining a posterior splint with the U splint gives added stability.
Foot	A pillow splint is excellent for emergency care. If splinting is necessary for an extended time, however, a posterior plaster slab combined with a U splint is usually best.

5

ORTHOPAEDIC EMERGENCIES

Douglas R. Dirschl

Few orthopaedic conditions are immediately life threatening. However, a significant number of orthopaedic conditions can threaten the viability of the injured limb if not recognized and treated within a few hours of injury. It is important to be able to recognize orthopaedic injuries that require emergent or urgent treatment and to distinguish them from those that require semi-elective treatment. The purpose of this chapter is to acquaint the reader with life-threatening and potentially limb-threatening orthopaedic conditions.

■ LIFE-THREATENING ORTHOPAEDIC CONDITIONS

Many patients with orthopaedic injuries are the victims of multiple trauma. As such, they may have numerous musculoskeletal and nonmusculoskeletal injuries. Although intraabdominal, intrathoracic, or intracranial injuries may be immediately life threatening, an open tibial fracture is only potentially limb threatening. Thus every patient with orthopaedic injuries should be evaluated for signs of life-threatening, nonmusculoskeletal injuries, which require emergent management.

Unstable Fractures of the Pelvis

Unstable fractures of the pelvis can result in a threefold increase in the intrapelvic volume. These fractures can disrupt the pelvic veins, which lie along the inside of the posterior pelvis, and the subsequent hemorrhage into the enlarged pelvic cavity can result in profound shock and even death. Immediate recognition of the patient with an unstable fracture of the pelvis and hypovolemic shock is critical to preserving the patient's life. Although it is beyond the scope of this text to discuss the causes and definitive treatment of unstable fractures of the pelvis, it is important to remember that all patients sustaining high-energy orthopaedic trauma (such as motor vehicle crashes) should have an AP pelvic radiograph made in the first few minutes after arrival in the emergency department. Examination of an AP radiograph of the pelvis is all that is required to diagnose an unstable fracture of the pelvis.

In a patient with an unstable fracture of the pelvis and hypovolemic shock, immediate compression and stabilization of the pelvis is necessary. Ideally, this is done with an external skeletal fixator applied in the emergency department trauma bay. In the absence of such a device, MAST trousers with the pelvic portion inflated can be used as a temporary measure. Finally, if nothing else is available, a sheet beneath the patient's pelvis can be pulled over his abdomen and tied tightly in a knot to form a "pelvic sling" and slow hemorrhage in the pelvis.

■ POTENTIALLY LIMB-THREATENING ORTHOPAEDIC INJURIES

Arterial Injury

Although the peripheral arteries normally are not considered part of the musculoskeletal system, arterial injuries warrant inclusion here because fractures, dislocations, and crushing injuries of the limbs can disrupt the vascular system. Classic findings in an arterial disruption are a pale, cold, asensate, pulseless limb. More commonly, however, sensory loss may be the only early indication of vascular compromise. Since the appearance of classic clinical signs is often delayed, the physician must maintain a high index of suspicion for arterial injury in all patients sustaining orthopaedic injuries, especially those occurring near an artery. Orthopaedic and vascular surgeons should be consulted in all cases of suspected arterial injury associated with a fracture or dislocation.

Traumatic Amputation

Traumatic amputation of the fingertips, usually the result of an accident with a power saw, are commonly seen in hospital emergency departments and are usually managed with wound debridement and closure. Amputations of entire fingers, hands, arms, or lower limbs are much less common but are devastating injuries and should prompt *immediate* orthopaedic consultation. The possibility of replantation should be considered in all patients with traumatic amputations. In general, the more distal the injury and the shorter the time from injury to surgery, the greater the chance for successful replantation of the amputated part. Replantation is also more likely to succeed in a child and in a clean amputation with little or no crushing or avulsion. The most commonly replanted parts are fingers, especially the index finger and thumb. In adults, replantation of traumatic amputations in the lower extremity are rarely attempted because of the poor functional results.

The physician should apply a sterile compression dressing to control hemorrhage from the residual limb; a tourniquet should be applied only if compression is unsuccessful. The amputated part should be preserved by wrapping it in sterile gauze moistened with cool Ringer's lactate or normal saline solution and sealing it in a clean, dry container. The part should not be exposed directly to ice but may be placed in ice water.

Compartment Syndrome

Increased pressure within a closed fascial compartment can obstruct the microcirculation to the nerves and muscles lying within and distal to the involved space, leading to tissue necrosis, which can be irreversible after 4 to 6 hours. Such increased pressure can result from hemorrhage or edema associated with acute injury, sustained external pressure on a limb, or muscular overexertion. Constricting casts, dressings, and splints can also increase compartmental pressures.

The classic signs of compartment syndromes are the *five Ps:* paresthesias, pallor, pulselessness, pain out of proportion to the injury, and pain on passive stretch.

Severe ischemic pain is the most prominent finding in the alert patient with acute compartment syndrome. The pain is generally believed by the treating nurse and physician to be out of proportion to the injury the patient sustained. The involved compartments are generally swollen and may be very tight. Passive stretch of ischemic muscle is painful and is the most sensitive sign of developing compartment syndrome. Local injury can cause stretch pain without ischemia, however. Peripheral nerves are sensitive to ischemia, and progressive loss of sensory and motor function—often preceded by paresthesia—is a reliable early sign of compartment syndrome. Normal sensory and motor function of all the local nerves is rare if significant compartment syndrome is present at the time of examination. Pallor, that is, capillary refill time longer than 4 seconds in the injured digits, and pulselessness are late signs of compartment syndrome and should not be relied on heavily to make the early diagnosis.

Compartment syndrome is treated initially by releasing any constricting casts, splints, or dressings. If symptoms persist, orthopaedic consultation should be obtained for measurement of compartmental pressures and consideration for operative fasciotomy. Compartment syndrome is discussed in greater detail in Chapter 32.

Open Fractures

Any break in the skin that communicates with a fracture and its hematoma permits bacterial contamination of the bone, which generally has poor resistance to infection. A variety of complications can result from open fractures, even if the open wound is only a small puncture. Open pelvic fractures are especially dangerous, with a mortality rate approaching 50%.

When in doubt, assume that any nearby skin wound communicates with the underlying fracture. Limited exploration and probing of wounds in the emergency department cannot reliably rule out an open fracture. In cases of open fracture a sterile dressing should be applied over the open wound, the extremity splinted, and immediate orthopaedic consultation obtained.

Dislocation of the Knee

Dislocation of the knee is a rare injury, usually the result of high-energy trauma, most commonly when a pedestrian is struck by a motor vehicle. In the most common direction of dislocation, the tibia moves posterior to the distal femur. Such an anatomic alignment puts great stress on the popliteal artery and the posterior tibial and peroneal nerves; in fact, the incidence of arterial and neurologic injury following posterior dislocation of the knee is high. Patients with posterior dislocation of the knee should be carefully examined for neurologic dysfunction. The dislocation should be immediately reduced and the knee splinted, followed by a second neurologic examination. Although the recommendation is somewhat controversial, many authors recommend that an arteriogram of the popliteal artery be obtained for all patients sustaining a knee dislocation regardless of their vascular status on clinical examination following reduction of the dislocation.

Dislocation of the Hip

Traumatic dislocation of the hip generally occurs when the flexed hip is forced posteriorly out of the acetabulum, as can occur when the knee strikes the dashboard in a head-on motor vehicle collision. The hip is generally held in a flexed, internally rotated, and adducted position, and any motion of the hip is extremely painful. Radiographs will clearly reveal the dislocation and often a fracture of the posterior wall of the acetabulum or femoral head. Orthopaedic consultation should be obtained immediately, since the outcome following posterior dislocation of the hip is much worse if the hip is not reduced within the first 6 hours following injury.

Fracture of the Femoral Neck in a Young Adult

Femoral neck fractures occur commonly in the osteoporotic elderly population, most often because of a simple fall. Femoral neck fractures in young adults occur rarely and are almost always the result of high-energy trauma. A femoral neck fracture in a child or young adult is considered an orthopaedic emergency. High-energy femoral neck fractures can easily disrupt the tenuous arterial blood supply to the femoral head, and early reduction and stabilization of these fractures may offer the only chance for restoring blood flow to the femoral head and preventing the dreaded complication of avascular necrosis. Immediate orthopaedic consultation should be sought in any child or young adult patient with a fracture of the femoral neck.

PATIENT-RELATED
PROBLEMS

PROBLEMS WITHOUT ASSOCIATED TRAUMA (OVERUSE AND DEGENERATIVE CONDITIONS)

□ 6 □

NECK PAIN

Douglas R. Dirschl

Degeneration of cervical intervertebral disks is a nearly universal finding in adult patients and may result in arthritis (spondylosis) or in protrusion of part of the disk contents (herniated nucleus pulposus). These two degenerative conditions cause most of the nontraumatic disorders of the neck encountered in orthopaedic practice. The physician must keep in mind that disorders or tumors of nonmusculoskeletal structures in the neck can also be a source of neck pain.

■ PHONE CALL

Questions

1. **How long has the pain been present?**
   The sudden onset of severe neck pain may indicate an acute strain, sudden disk herniation, or, in rare cases, subluxation of the cervical vertebrae. Neck pain present for weeks or months generally indicates an arthritic condition.
2. **Does the pain radiate to the fingers? Does the patient complain of any numbness or tingling in the fingers?**
   Pain, numbness, tingling, or electric shock sensations radiating to the fingers may indicate inflammation or impingement of cervical nerve roots in the neck, often due to a herniated cervical disk.
3. **Has the patient sustained any trauma to the neck?**
   In the absence of trauma a fracture of a cervical vertebra or a cervical strain (whiplash) is unlikely. The evaluation and management of neck pain in the presence of a traumatic injury is discussed in Chapter 21.

Orders

None.

Inform RN

"I will arrive at the bedside/emergency department in 30 to 60 minutes." In general, nearly all patients with neck pain not associated with a traumatic injury do not require urgent evaluation. If the patient complains of numbness or tingling in the fingers, however, there might be an associated neurologic problem, and the patient should be evaluated more urgently.

■ ELEVATOR THOUGHTS

- Arthritis/arthrosis
  Spondylosis (osteoarthritis)
  Herniated cervical disk
  Spondylolisthesis
  Rheumatoid arthritis
  Ankylosing spondylitis
- Infections of bone
  Pyogenic osteomyelitis
  Tuberculous osteomyelitis
  Paravertebral abscess
- Deformities
  Torticollis (wry neck)
  Congenital high scapula
  Sprengel's deformity
- Tumors
  Benign and malignant tumors of the neck or cervical spine
- Miscellaneous
  Cervical strain
  Fibromyositis

■ BEDSIDE

Vital Signs

Although the vital signs in the patient complaining of neck pain in the absence of trauma will likely be normal, they should be obtained anyway. Infection, tumor, and nonmusculoskeletal sources of neck pain may elicit abnormal vital signs. Special attention should also be given to performing a careful vascular examination in both upper limbs to ensure that vascular inflow is not impaired by whatever is causing the neck pain.

Selective History

Has there been any previous injury to or disorder of the neck?
It is important to ascertain the relationship of the present symptoms to any previous neck disorder. In most instances the cause of the neck pain will be the same as the cause of the prior neck pain.

Is there a history of stiffness of the neck?

Limitation in range of motion of the neck is a common feature in early stages of spondylosis or herniated cervical disk.

Does the pain remain in the neck, or does it radiate to other areas?

It is important to determine the pattern of radiation of the pain and whether the pain is related to any particular movements or positions. Pain extending to the arms and fingers is likely caused by inflammation of or pressure on a nerve root in the cervical region. Pain caused by pressure on a nerve such as this follows a clearly defined course that depends entirely on the dermatome distribution of the nerve root involved (Fig. 6–1).

What other medical problems does the patient have?

A history of rheumatoid arthritis or Down's syndrome should lead the physician to consider cervical instability as a cause of the symptoms, whereas a history of ankylosing spondylitis should prompt the physician to suspect spontaneous fracture through the ankylosed vertebrae.

Selective Physical Examination

Inspection

It is essential to observe the disrobed patient from the front and back to assess the contours of the soft tissues as well as the bones about the neck and shoulder. Localized swelling of the anterior neck may indicate a tumor, abscess, or other nonmusculoskeletal source for the pain. A high-riding scapula or webbing of the neck may indicate a congenital spinal condition, such as Sprengel's deformity. A rigid posture of the neck may indicate muscle spasm or ankylosis. The physician should also look for previous scars, open wounds, or draining sinuses.

Palpation

The physician should palpate gently, first assessing skin temperature throughout the neck. Localized warmth could be a sign of deep infection. The size and character of any areas of soft tissue swelling should be assessed. Localized tenderness should be sought and characterized as to its anatomic location. Tenderness overlying the sternocleidomastoid or trapezius muscle is common with neck strain but may also be seen with spondylosis or herniated cervical disk. Maximal tenderness directly over the spinous processes of the cervical vertebrae rarely is caused by strain, spondylosis, or herniated disk.

Movements

The physician should assess flexion and extension, lateral bending, and rotation of the cervical spine. Although pain may limit motion in all conditions, only in spondylosis, ankylosis, or deformity of the neck should motion be truly restricted. One should assess the character and location of pain associated with movement. Pain or tingling radiating to the fingers with motion of the neck (especially when the neck is turning to the contralateral side) may indicate impingement of a nerve root within the intervertebral foramina.

Neurologic Status of the Upper Limb

The physician should carefully examine the motor and sensory function of all peripheral nerves in both upper extremities. Dys-

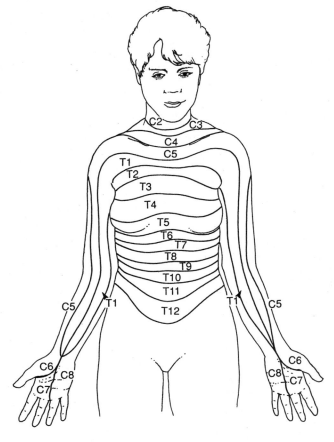

Figure 6–1 □ Dermatome distributions of the upper limb and trunk. (From Porterfield JA, DeRosa C: Mechanical Neck Pain: Perspectives in Functional Anatomy. Philadelphia, WB Saunders, 1995, p 148.)

Table 6–1 □ **TESTING OF CERVICAL NERVE ROOTS**

Root	Motor Function	Sensory Distribution	Reflex
C5	Deltoid muscle	Shoulder and lateral arm	Biceps
C6	Wrist extension	Lateral forearm and thumb	Brachioradialis
C7	Wrist flexion	Long finger	Triceps
C8	Finger flexion	Medial forearm and small finger	None
T1	Finger abduction	Medial arm	None

function in the distribution of a peripheral nerve is generally not related to cervical spine pathology but rather to pathology more distal in the arm or forearm. The physician should also assess the neurologic function in each nerve root distribution in the upper limb. The motor function, sensory distribution, and reflex for each of the cervical nerve roots is summarized in Table 6–1. Neurologic impairment confined to a single nerve root level generally is due to impingement of the nerve root at the level of the cervical spine.

Further Orders

It is wise to obtain a cervical spine series of radiographs in most patients complaining of spontaneous or increasing neck pain. This series of radiographs consists of AP, lateral, oblique, and odontoid views. In patients known to have rheumatoid arthritis, ankylosing spondylitis, or Down's syndrome, flexion and extension lateral radiographs may also be of assistance in assessing stability of the spine. *Flexion and extension radiographs should be obtained, however, only after the standard cervical spine series has been reviewed and found to be normal; flexion and extension of an unstable neck could be dangerous.*

■ MANAGEMENT

Since most causes of neck pain in the absence of trauma are due to degenerative changes, definitive treatment is usually symptomatic. Most patients should be prescribed NSAIDs, whereas those with muscle spasm may receive mild antispasmodics. In general, nonsedating antispasmodics, such as metaxalone (Skelaxin) are preferred over antispasmodics with strong sedative effects (e.g., diazepam [Valium] and cyclobenzaprine [Flexeril]). Narcotic analgesics generally are not recommended for patients with neck pain due to strain or spondylosis; narcotics are not particularly effective in these conditions, and their use may result in dependency. Application of heat to the neck may alleviate symptoms.

The institution of a physical therapy protocol consisting of stretching exercises and modalities such as ultrasound and phonophoresis to the neck may also be of benefit. Use of a soft cervical collar for relief of symptoms is controversial; short-term use of the collar may relieve symptoms and will cause no harm, but prolonged use can weaken the cervical musculature and lead to reliance on the collar to control pain.

Patients with abnormalities on radiographs or on neurologic examination of the upper extremities should have an orthopaedic or neurosurgical consultation. The consultant will evaluate the patient and determine the need for any additional imaging studies, such as CT scanning, myelography, or MRI scanning.

7

SHOULDER PAIN

Douglas R. Dirschl

The mechanics of the shoulder are complex. The shoulder joint is actually three joints: the glenohumeral joint (the true shoulder joint), the acromioclavicular joint, and the sternoclavicular joint. In the normal shoulder, all three joints function together in the performance of daily activities. In addition, the glenohumeral joint is inherently unstable, relying on a fine balance of ligament and muscle stability to maintain it in a reduced position. Any imbalance of these finely tuned structures will result in pain about the shoulder.

■ PHONE CALL

Questions

1. **How long has the shoulder pain been present?**
   The sudden onset of severe shoulder pain may indicate infection, tendon rupture, or trauma. The insidious onset of pain or chronic pain may indicate a degenerative or overuse condition.
2. **Does the patient have a history of cardiac problems?**
   The pain associated with myocardial ischemia is frequently referred to the shoulder. The physician should be aware that many victims of myocardial infarction experience only shoulder pain, no chest pain.
3. **Does the pain radiate to the hand or fingers?**
   Referred pain from inflamed or irritated cervical nerve roots usually extends from the neck over the top of the shoulder and into the arm. Unlike true shoulder pain, it radiates below the elbow into the forearm.
4. **Has the patient sustained any trauma to the shoulder?**
   A traumatic injury to the shoulder can result in fracture, dislocation, or tendon rupture. Please see Chapter 22 for a discussion of the evaluation and management of shoulder pain associated with trauma.

Orders

None.

Inform RN

"I will arrive at the bedside/emergency department in 30 to 60 minutes." In the absence of cardiac dysfunction, pain in the shoulder without traumatic injury is rarely urgent and does not require immediate evaluation.

■ ELEVATOR THOUGHTS

Disorders of the Glenohumeral Joint
- Arthritis / arthrosis
  Pyogenic arthritis
  Tuberculous arthritis
  Rheumatoid arthritis
  Osteoarthrosis
  Arthrofibrosis (frozen shoulder, adhesive capsulitis)
- Mechanical derangement
  Dislocation
  Complete tear of the rotator cuff
  Impingement syndrome
  Rupture of the long head of the biceps
  Internal derangement

Disorders of the Acromioclavicular Joint
- Osteoarthrosis
- Dislocation or subluxation
- Osteolysis of the distal clavicle

Disorders of the Sternoclavicular Joint
- Arthrosis
- Persistent or recurrent dislocation

■ BEDSIDE

Vital Signs

Because the pain of myocardial ischemia can be referred to the shoulder, vital signs should be obtained in patients with sudden, spontaneous shoulder pain in the absence of trauma.

Selective History

What is the precise location and distribution of the pain?
True shoulder pain is seldom confined to the shoulder itself. Typically, it radiates from a point near the tip of the acromion down the lateral side of the arm to the level of the deltoid muscle insertion. It is unusual for true shoulder pain to radiate below the elbow. Pain arising in the acromioclavicular joint or sternoclavicular joint is usually localized to the joint itself and does not radiate down the limb.

Does the patient have a history of previous shoulder injury or dysfunction?

It is important to assess whether the patient has any prior history of shoulder dysfunction, such as rotator cuff tendinitis, previous dislocation, or prior surgery. The most common cause of recurrent shoulder pain is the same entity that caused the prior episode of shoulder pain.

Does the shoulder lock or catch?

True locking of the shoulder, with the joint frozen and incapable of active or passive motion, is rare and may indicate an intraarticular derangement or loose body. Catching of the shoulder is common and, although the physician should suspect an intraarticular disorder, may be associated with both intraarticular and extraarticular pathology.

What activities can the patient perform with the involved arm?

The impact of the condition on the patient's activities of daily living should be assessed. The physician should ask if the patient can reach overhead or perform other common activities, such as combing the hair or brushing the teeth.

What activities or movements bring on the pain?

Constant, boring pain in the shoulder likely is caused by a different injury or disorder than is pain that is apparent only after lifting 50 lb (22.5 kg) boxes for 8 hours. Constant pain is generally related to an acute injury or inflammatory condition, whereas pain after activity generally indicates an overuse condition.

Selective Physical Examination

Inspection

Begin the examination from behind the disrobed patient and inspect the contours of the bones and soft tissues of the shoulder, comparing always with the contralateral side. Alteration of the normal bony contours may indicate dislocation of a joint, whereas muscular atrophy may be indicative of a rotator cuff disruption or neurologic injury. Acromioclavicular separation is easily identified by the prominence of the distal clavicle on the involved side. Localized swelling and erythema may indicate infection or tumor.

Palpation

The skin should be palpated for localized areas of warmth, which might indicate deep infection. The bones and soft tissue should be palpated for specific sites of tenderness. Areas of tenderness should be carefully related to the underlying anatomic structures, as this is the simplest way to diagnose most orthopaedic conditions about the shoulder. For example, tenderness over the acromioclavicular joint almost always indicates a mild acromioclavicular separation or degenerative disease of that joint, and tenderness at the anterolateral corner of the acromion usually indicates impingement syndrome. In the shoulder, as in all areas of the musculoskeletal system, a thorough knowledge of the functional anatomy is essential to making the correct diagnosis in most situations.

Movements

While observing from behind, have the seated patient abduct both arms from the sides as far as possible. Look not only to determine the range of motion but also to see if the scapulae move smoothly and symmetrically along the thorax throughout the range of movement. Asymmetric motion of the scapulae may indicate fibrosis or neurologic dysfunction. Pain with movement and its location should also be sought. One should gently palpate the entire shoulder region for crepitus while the patient moves in flexion and extension and internal and external rotation. Crepitus in the area of the anterior acromion or bicipital groove may indicate fibrosis, tendinitis, or the presence of calcium deposits.

Neurologic Examination

The physician should test the strength of the shoulder in elevation, abduction, extension, internal and external rotation, and in retraction and protraction of the scapula. Sensibility should also be tested, especially over the lateral aspect of the shoulder, where the sensory distribution of the axillary nerve is located.

Examination of Specific Areas

Acromioclavicular Joint

The acromioclavicular joint should be palpated for swelling, warmth, or tenderness. Crossing the symptomatic arm across the patient's chest is one way of compressing the acromioclavicular joint; pain on this motion may be indicative of acromioclavicular arthritis.

Sternoclavicular Joint

The sternoclavicular area should be palpated for swelling, increased warmth, and tenderness. Tenderness at this joint may indicate arthritis or unreduced dislocation.

Glenohumeral Joint

Full range of motion in internal and external rotation generally indicates that the glenohumeral joint is not dislocated. Tenderness at the anterolateral border of the acromion generally indicates bursitis or rotator cuff tendinitis, both of which are more appropriately referred to as impingement syndrome. A further test for impingement syndrome involves having the patient abduct the arm 90 degrees and internally rotate the arm so the thumb points downward. Pain on this movement is generally indicative of inflammation along the insertion of the rotator cuff into the greater tuberosity.

Further Orders

Any patient with suspected infection or dislocation and nearly every patient with shoulder pain should be referred for radiographs of the shoulder. A shoulder series includes AP views in both internal and external rotation, as well as an axillary view. All three views are necessary to adequately evaluate the shoulder. Although other special views have been described, they are rarely necessary in the initial evaluation of the patient with shoulder pain.

■ MANAGEMENT

With the exception of infection and dislocation, atraumatic conditions of the shoulders rarely require emergency management. Immediate orthopaedic consultation should be obtained for all suspected dislocations or infections of the shoulder, and elective orthopaedic consultation should be obtained in nearly all other cases of shoulder pain. Treatment mainstays for inflammatory conditions of the shoulder, such as impingement syndrome, are NSAIDs and specific strengthening exercises. The most important muscles to strengthen are those of the rotator cuff, particularly the supraspinatus and infraspinatus. Referral to a physical therapist for instruction in these strengthening exercises may be helpful. In general, movement of the shoulder is encouraged for all conditions; a sling, if used at all, should be used only to enhance comfort for a short time; long-term use of an arm sling may lead to stiffness of the shoulder and elbow.

Any condition involving stiffness of the shoulder should be managed immediately with referral to a physical therapist for aggressive range of motion exercises of the shoulder. Frozen shoulder, or idiopathic arthrofibrosis of the shoulder, most commonly occurs in women over 50 years of age and may have a protracted course. Aggressive and persistent physical therapy for range of motion exercises usually will improve motion, but maximal improvement may not be realized for more than a year. Patients with a frozen shoulder that is refractory to 3 to 6 months of aggressive physical therapy should be referred to an orthopaedist for consideration for shoulder manipulation and arthroscopic lysis of adhesions.

Although injections are frequently used for rotator cuff tendinitis and impingement syndrome, they probably are not indicated as the initial treatment and should be performed only if NSAIDs and physical therapy do not relieve symptoms. Physical therapy for patients with impingement syndrome should consist of rotator cuff stretching and strengthening exercises, focusing on the supraspinatus and infraspinatus muscles.

Acromioclavicular and sternoclavicular disease is treated with NSAIDs, range of motion exercises, and observation. Local injections of corticosteroid preparations can also be helpful. If symptoms are not relieved in 6 weeks, the patient should be referred to an orthopaedist for consideration of operative treatment.

True internal derangement of the shoulder can be difficult to diagnose on physical examination alone. Patients usually will complain of locking or catching of the shoulder, often only in a certain position. Patients with suspected internal derangement of the shoulder should be referred to an orthopaedic specialist for further evaluation and treatment.

8

ARM AND ELBOW PAIN

Douglas R. Dirschl

Apart from traumatic injury, disorders of the arm and elbow are generally straightforward and present few diagnostic or management problems. The elbow, although not particularly prone to osteoarthritis, is second only to the knee in the incidence of osteochondritis dissecans and loose body formation. The ulnar nerve lies in a vulnerable position behind the medial epicondyle, and the possibility of impairment of ulnar nerve function should always be remembered.

■ PHONE CALL

Questions

1. **How long has the pain been present?**

   The sudden onset of severe pain may indicate an injury, infection, or sudden mechanical derangement of the elbow, whereas the insidious onset of pain usually indicates a degenerative or overuse condition.

2. **Does the pain radiate to the hand?**

   Pain originating from the bones or muscles in the arm or elbow seldom radiates to the hand. Pain from irritation of the ulnar nerve, however, will radiate to the ring and small fingers.

3. **Does the patient have a previous history of arm or elbow problems?**

   The most common cause of elbow or arm pain in a patient with a previous history of such pain is the same condition that caused the previous arm or elbow pain.

4. **Does the patient complain of any locking or catching of the elbow?**

   Locking of the elbow (sudden, intermittent inability to extend or flex the elbow) is a typical sign of a loose body in the elbow.

Orders

None.

Inform RN

"I will arrive at the bedside/emergency department in 30 to 60 minutes." In the absence of deformity, trauma, infection, or progressive neurologic dysfunction, pain in the arm and elbow does not require urgent evaluation.

■ ELEVATOR THOUGHTS

Disorders of the Arm
- Acute and chronic osteomyelitis
- Tumors
  - Benign tumors of bone
  - Malignant tumors of bone

Disorders of the Elbow
- Arthritis/arthrosis
  - Pyogenic arthritis
  - Rheumatoid arthritis
  - Tuberculous arthritis
  - Osteoarthrosis
  - Hemophilic arthritis
- Mechanical derangement
  - Osteochondritis dissecans
  - Loose bodies in the elbow
- Deformities
  - Cubitus valgus
  - Cubitus varus
- Extraarticular disorders
  - Lateral epicondylitis (tennis elbow)
  - Olecranon bursitis
  - Ulnar nerve entrapment at the cubital tunnel

■ BEDSIDE

Vital Signs

Vital signs are generally not necessary in patients with atraumatic pain in the upper arm and elbow. If, however, infection of the arm or elbow is suspected, the patient's vital signs should be obtained.

Selective History

What is the specific location of the pain and does the pain radiate anywhere?

It is important to ascertain the exact location and distribution of the pain, as well as its nature. Pain arising locally in the arm is easily confused with pain arising in the shoulder, which characteristically radiates to a point about halfway down the outer aspect of the arm. Elbow pain is generally localized precisely to the joint, although a diffuse aching pain can also be felt in the forearm. If the ulnar nerve is entrapped in the cubital tunnel behind the medial epicondyle, pain and paresthesias can occur on the ulnar side of the hand.

Is the pain continuous or intermittent? Is it associated with particular activities?

Continuous pain generally indicates an acute inflammatory process in the region. The physician should keep in mind that acute inflammation can be due to infection, injury, strain, or tumor. Pain occurring with activity is the general rule in the arm and elbow. Arthritic conditions are generally painful on motion or stress of the involved joints, whereas mechanical derangement or loose body formation within a joint is characterized by intermittent, severe pain with use of the joint.

Does the patient have a prior history of elbow injury or disorder?

In the elbow a history of previous injury is often significant. Injuries in this area can frequently have late effects in the form of impaired movement, deformity, loose body formation, or entrapment of the ulnar nerve. If the previous elbow injury occurred when the patient was a child, growth disturbances may have resulted in cubitus varus or valgus.

Selective Physical Examination

Inspection

One should inspect both arms and elbows simultaneously, comparing the contours of the soft tissues and bones. Localized swelling may indicate an infection or a tumor. Comparison of the bony alignment with the contralateral elbow may also be helpful. Increased varus or valgus at the elbow may be indicative of an old fracture with malunion or a disturbance of growth.

Palpation

Skin temperature should be assessed. Areas of warmth may indicate infection, tumor, or inflammatory arthritis of the elbow. Local tenderness should be sought, and its precise location should be assessed in relation to the anatomic structures lying directly beneath the palpating finger. Tenderness over the humerus itself may indicate infection or tumor, whereas tenderness directly over the olecranon or lateral epicondyle of the humerus may indicate olecranon bursitis and lateral epicondylitis, respectively. Fullness on the lateral side of the elbow just anterior to the olecranon is indicative of an elbow effusion. This sign, although nonspecific, should prompt the physician to search carefully for a fracture or another acute injury.

Movements

The humeroulnar joint should be tested for active and passive flexion and extension and compared with these movements on the contralateral side. Movements of the radioulnar and radiohumeral joints should be assessed by comparing active and passive pronation and supination with these movements on the contralateral side. Pain or crepitation on movement should also be noted and may indicate intraarticular pathology. Painless limitation of movement is usually indicative of a chronic degenerative condition, such as osteoarthrosis.

Stability

The physician should stress the extended elbow of the relaxed patient into varus and valgus, searching for pain and instability not found on the contralateral side. If lateral epicondylitis is suspected and the patient is tender over the lateral humeral epicondyle, extension of the elbow and flexion of the wrist and fingers may reproduce the pain. This position places the common extensor muscle origin (the location of inflammation in tennis elbow) on maximal stress and may reproduce the patient's symptoms.

Ulnar Nerve

Sensory function of the ulnar nerve is assessed by evaluating the sensibility over the ulnar surface of the dorsum of the hand, as well as the volar surface of the small and ring fingers. Motor function in the ulnar nerve is assessed by testing the flexor digitorum profundus muscles as well as the interosseous muscles in the hand. Tinel's sign may be elicited by lightly tapping over the ulnar nerve behind the medial epicondyle and asking the patient if he or she feels a shooting or tingling sensation in the fingertips. Firm tapping is to be avoided, as all patients will have tingling in the fingers with firm tapping over the ulnar nerve at the elbow.

Further Orders

Radiographs of the arm and elbow should be obtained in all patients with pain in this area to further assess the region. Osteomyelitis or tumors of bone may be seen on plain radiographs. Loose bodies or arthritis of the elbow can also be visualized on AP and true lateral radiographs of the elbow. If infection is suspected, a complete blood count (CBC) and erythrocyte sedimentation rate (ESR) should be obtained.

■ MANAGEMENT

Aside from infection and tumor, most atraumatic conditions causing pain in the arm and elbow do not require urgent management. If tumor or infection is suspected, orthopaedic consultation should be obtained immediately. Orthopaedic consultation should also be obtained for suspected loose bodies in the elbow, olecranon bursitis, lateral epicondylitis, or arthritis of the elbow, but consultation need not be urgent. General nonoperative management for elbow pain consists of range of motion exercises, administration of NSAIDs, compression wrapping, and occasional immobilization in an arm sling for comfort. An arm sling should not be used long term, as it definitely will lead to stiffness of the elbow.

Olecranon bursitis is treated with compression wrapping, activity modification to avoid excessive pressure over the region, and NSAIDs. If the patient's work requires him or her to rest frequently on the elbows and the job cannot be modified to reduce pressure on the area, consideration should be given to padding the elbow to prevent excessive pressure on the area. If symptoms do not resolve in 4 to 6 weeks, orthopaedic consultation should be sought. Infected olecranon bursitis is generally best treated with antibiotics and surgical excision of the infected bursa.

Nonoperative management for lateral epicondylitis is nearly always successful and consists of administration of NSAIDs, stretching exercises, icing, and activity modifications. Physical therapy and modalities such as ultrasound and phonophoresis are sometimes helpful. Stretching involves extension of the elbow combined with flexion of the wrist and fingers. Modification of activities to avoid those activities that exacerbate symptoms is important, as is icing the area before and after activity. Tennis elbow straps wrapped tightly around the proximal forearm can relieve stress on the lateral epicondyle and are often helpful. Injection of the area with corticosteroids can be helpful in patients refractory to the other treatment methods.

9

FOREARM AND WRIST PAIN

Douglas R. Dirschl

In the absence of acute or remote injury, isolated pain in the forearm and wrist is rare. Elbow pain occasionally may radiate to the forearm, and pain due to nerve compression within the forearm or wrist generally causes symptoms in the hands and the fingers (i.e., carpal tunnel syndrome). A thorough understanding of the anatomy of the muscles, bones, and nerves in the forearm is necessary for the accurate diagnosis of pain in the forearm and wrist.

■ PHONE CALL

Questions

1. **How long has the pain been present?**
   The sudden onset of severe pain generally indicates an acute inflammatory process, such as infection or acute strain, or an acute injury to the region. The slow, insidious onset of symptoms or symptoms present for weeks to months generally indicate a degenerative or overuse condition.
2. **Does the pain radiate to the hand or fingers?**
   Pain originating in the bones of the forearm or wrist or in the wrist joint itself rarely radiates to the fingers. Since the musculotendinous unit of the finger flexors and extensors extends from the proximal forearm to the fingertips, inflammation of this mechanism can result in pain extending throughout the forearm and fingers. Peripheral nerve entrapment in the forearm or wrist frequently results in pain, numbness, or tingling in the fingers.
3. **Has the patient sustained an injury recently?**
   Fracture, ligamentous injury, or acute strain or sprain are common about the wrist, often due to injury as minor as a fall from standing height. For additional information on the evaluation and management of forearm and wrist pain associated with trauma, see Chapter 24.

Orders

None.

Inform RN

"I will arrive at the bedside/emergency department in 30 to 60 minutes." In the absence of infection or major trauma, spontaneous pain in the forearm and wrist rarely requires urgent evaluation.

■ ELEVATOR THOUGHTS

Disorders of the Forearm
- Infections
  - Acute and chronic osteomyelitis
  - Abscess
- Tumors of bone and soft tissue
  - Benign tumors
  - Malignant tumors
- Miscellaneous
  - Acute tenosynovitis
  - Compartment syndrome
  - Volkmann's ischemic contracture

Disorders of the Wrist
- Arthritis/arthrosis
  - Pyogenic arthritis
  - Rheumatoid arthritis
  - Osteoarthrosis
- Deformities
  - Madelung's deformity
- Miscellaneous
  - Kienböck disease
  - Carpal instability
  - Ganglion cyst
  - De Quervain's tenovaginitis (sometimes referred to as tenosynovitis)
  - Acute tenosynovitis

■ BEDSIDE

Vital Signs

In the absence of major trauma, vital signs are rarely necessary for evaluation of spontaneous pain in the forearm and wrist. If infection is suspected, however, the patient's temperature should be obtained.

Selective History

What is the precise location of the pain, and where does the pain radiate?

The precise location and character of the pain should be assessed, as well as its radiation to any other area. The physician must remember that symptoms in the hand and wrist can be caused by impingement of a cervical nerve root in the neck. Inquiries should always be made about previous neck or upper extremity disorders or injuries.

Has the patient recently increased use of the extremity?

Since most pain in the forearm and wrist in the absence of trauma is related to overuse, the patient should be questioned about any recent overuse or unusual activities.

Selective Physical Examination

Inspection

Both forearms and wrists should be inspected simultaneously, and comparison should be made to the contralateral forearm to identify any alterations in the soft tissue or bony contours. Localized swelling and erythema may indicate abscess or tumor, whereas generalized swelling may indicate compartment syndrome. Localized swelling over the dorsum of the wrist may indicate acute tenosynovitis. A ganglion cyst is often seen as a firm localized mass apparent on the dorsum of the wrist.

Palpation

The skin should be palpated for warmth, which if present may indicate infection, tumor, or tenosynovitis. Areas of local tenderness should be identified and related to the specific anatomic structures beneath the palpating finger. Special attention should be paid to palpation of the bony prominences and extensor tendon sheaths at the wrist. Bone tenderness may indicate fracture or osteomyelitis, and tenderness and fullness over the extensor tendons generally indicates tenosynovitis. A firm, nontender, mobile, well-defined mass over the dorsum of the wrist is the usual finding in a ganglion cyst of the wrist. The cyst is felt more easily when the wrist is flexed and may be so firm the examiner mistakes it for a displaced carpal bone. Tenderness over the radial styloid and along the course of the abductor tendons of the thumb may indicate de Quervain's tenovaginitis.

Movements

Active and passive movements at the wrist should be assessed, including flexion and extension of the wrist, radial and ulnar deviation of the wrist, and supination and pronation of the forearm. The examiner should specifically search for limitations of motion or pain with range of motion. As always, the location of the pain should be sought.

Neurologic Examination

The power of each muscle group in control of wrist and finger movement should be ascertained. Sensibility testing should also be performed over the forearm and hand.

Special Tests

Finkelstein's test for stenosing tenosynovitis of the extensor tendons to the thumb (de Quervain's tenovaginitis) is performed by having the patient gently make a fist with the thumb inside the fingers. The wrist is then moved into ulnar deviation. Acute pain along the course of the abductor pollicis longus tendon at the radial styloid constitutes a positive test result.

Further Orders

Patients presenting with pain in the forearm and wrist should have radiographs made to assess for any bony abnormalities or calcifications in the soft tissues. Soft tissue calcifications can occur with tumors or some types of tendinitis. The standard radiographic series of the forearm includes AP and lateral views. It is important to include both the wrist and elbow joints in the radiographs because, since the radius and ulna function as an interconnected unit, injury or lesion at either end of either bone may affect overall forearm and wrist function. The standard radiographic series of the wrist includes AP, oblique, and lateral views. All three views are necessary for the accurate diagnosis of wrist pathology. If infection of the forearm or wrist is suspected, a CBC and ESR should be obtained.

■ MANAGEMENT

With the exceptions of tumor and infection, the management of pain in the forearm and wrist in the absence of trauma is usually nonurgent. Management is generally symptomatic, including NSAIDs, compressive dressings as needed for comfort, and immobilization of the wrist as necessary to alleviate symptoms. A hand therapist can be helpful in mobilizing the soft tissues, reducing swelling, and enhancing joint mobility.

A ganglion cyst on the dorsum of the wrist is the most common benign soft tissue tumor in the musculoskeletal system. While the cyst does not require urgent treatment, the patient should be referred to an orthopaedist for discussion of treatment options, including potential surgical excision. Nonoperative treatment of ganglion cysts, generally consisting of aspiration with a large bore needle with or without injection of corticosteroids, results in disappearance of the cyst in about 50% of cases. Persistent pain and limitation of wrist function are the most common indications for surgical excision, but asymptomatic ganglions are occasionally excised for cosmetic reasons.

De Quervain's tenovaginitis is a common disorder affecting the abductor pollicis longus tendon as it passes through a tight fibro-osseous sheath over the radial styloid. Initial treatment consists of NSAIDs, range of motion exercises, modification of activities, and protection in a thumb spica splint. The proper position in which to immobilize the thumb is determined by having the patient gently oppose the thumb, index, and long fingers. Patients failing to respond to these treatment modalities in 4 to 6 weeks should be referred to an orthopaedist for further treatment, including consideration for surgical release of the tight sheath at the radial styloid.

Tenosynovitis of the extensor tendons as they pass over the dorsum of the wrist is common and may involve only a single tendon (the extensor carpi radialis is most common) or all of the tendons. Causes of this condition include overuse, repetitive motion, inflammatory arthritis, and metabolic disturbances (e.g., hypertension, pregnancy, diabetes, and hypothyroidism). Management is directed at reducing pain and swelling and promoting motion and usually includes NSAIDs, protective splints, and occupational therapy to help decrease edema and promote motion.

10

HAND AND FINGER PAIN

Douglas R. Dirschl

Many of the activities of everyday life depend on the efficient and smooth functioning of the hand. Because of the functional and economic consequences of hand disablement, care of the diseased or injured hand has become one of the most vital branches of orthopaedics. The physician must always remember that the hand does not tolerate immobilization well. The hand and fingers should be immobilized only when it is absolutely necessary to maintain stability following fractures or dislocations. The hand and fingers should be allowed free motion as soon as it is safe to do so; immobilization of the hand and fingers solely for the relief of pain generally should not be done.

■ PHONE CALLS

Questions

1. **How long has the pain been present?**
   The sudden onset of severe pain in the hand and fingers generally indicates infection or injury, whereas chronic pain generally indicates a degenerative or overuse condition.
2. **What is the specific location of the pain?**
   Knowing the specific location of the pain in the hand or fingers can be helpful in making the correct diagnosis. For example, pain around the fingernail is almost always due to inflammation or infection of the cuticle (eponychium), whereas pain at the base of the thumb most commonly is due to degenerative arthritis of the thumb carpometacarpal joint.
3. **Does the patient complain of numbness or tingling in the fingers?**
   Numbness or tingling usually indicates peripheral nerve compression, but tingling in the fingers does not localize the site of nerve compression to the hand; compression of a cervical nerve root or peripheral nerve anywhere from the neck to the fingertips can produce numbness and tingling in the fingers.
4. **Has this patient sustained an injury to the hand?**
   See Chapter 25 for a discussion of the evaluation and management of the injured hand.
5. **Does the patient have a history of injury to or disorder of the hand?**
   Knowledge of any prior injuries or disorders of the hand

and fingers is important to making the diagnosis. For example, malunited fractures of the scaphoid frequently are associated with a late onset of carpal instability and arthritis, and Dupuytren's contracture of the palmar fascia frequently recurs, even after surgical treatment.

Orders

None.

Inform RN

"I will arrive at the bedside/emergency department in 30 to 60 minutes." In the absence of infection or trauma, urgent evaluation of the patient with spontaneous pain in the hand and fingers is usually not necessary.

■ ELEVATOR THOUGHTS

- Infections
    - Acute infection of the fascial spaces in the palm
    - Pyogenic tenosynovitis
- Tumors of bone and soft tissues
- Neurologic disorders
    - Compression of the median nerve in the carpal tunnel
    - Compression of the ulnar nerve at the wrist
- Miscellaneous
    - Dupuytren's contracture
    - Rupture of tendons
    - Tenosynovitis
- Arthritis/arthrosis
    - Basilar thumb arthritis
    - Rheumatoid arthritis
    - Septic arthritis
    - Gouty arthritis

■ BEDSIDE

Vital Signs

In the absence of suspected infection, vital signs are not required in the evaluation of pain in the hand and fingers. If, however, infection is suspected, the patient's temperature should be obtained.

Selective History

What is the precise location of the pain?

As always, the physician must ascertain the specific location and the character of the pain. Burning pain at night waking the patient from sleep generally indicates nerve compression, whereas dull aching pain in the morning or with cold weather generally indicates degenerative arthritis. Localization of the aching pain to the base of the thumb may indicate basilar thumb arthritis.

How long have symptoms been present?
The time course of development of the pain should also be ascertained; slow, insidious onset of pain usually indicates an overuse or degenerative condition, whereas sudden onset of pain is indicative of an acute injury or an acute infectious or inflammatory process.

Does the patient have a history of problems with the hand and fingers?
Knowledge of any previous injuries, conditions, or surgeries in the painful area is a great help in making a diagnosis. For example, a history of inflammatory arthritis or gout may raise suspicion as to these disorders as a potential source for the hand and finger symptoms.

Selective Physical Examination

Inspection
The physician should inspect the affected hand and compare it to the contralateral hand. Specific notation should be made of the extent and location of swelling and erythema. Localized swelling or erythema usually indicates an infection of the hand but may also indicate a tumor. The resting posture of the hand should be ascertained and compared to that of the contralateral hand. Abnormal extension of a finger from the normal resting posture may indicate a flexor tendon rupture. Any deformity of the hand or fingers should be noted. Clawing of the small and ring fingers may indicate an injury to the ulnar nerve, whereas ulnar deviation of the fingers at the metacarpophalangeal (MCP) joints is a characteristic finding in rheumatoid arthritis. Hard, bandlike thickenings in the palm, sometimes associated with flexion deformities of the fingers, are characteristic for Dupuytren's contracture.

Palpation
The skin and soft tissues should be palpated for warmth as well as for local tenderness. Elevated temperature is generally indicative of infection or inflammatory synovitis. The location of tenderness should be ascertained and related to the anatomical structures beneath the palpating fingers. Tenderness at the base of the thumb may indicate basilar thumb arthritis, whereas a firm, tender mass in the pulp of a fingertip may indicate a soft tissue tumor (usually an epidermoid inclusion cyst or a giant cell tumor of tendon sheath—both benign). A firm mass or cord in the palm or fingers

restricting finger extension usually indicates Dupuytren's contracture, a benign but progressive contracture, and thickening of the palmar fascia.

Movements

Passive and active flexion and extension of all three joints of each finger should be ascertained. Asking the patient to make a fist is a simple way of testing active motion, and a simple way to quantify active motion is to measure the distance from the fingertips to the distal palmar crease on maximal flexion. Extension can easily be tested by asking the patient to extend the fingers. Passive motion is assessed by individually manipulating each joint in each finger.

Neurovascular Function

Careful assessment of sensory and motor function in the distributions of the median, ulnar, and radial nerves is vital to the evaluation of the hand and fingers (Fig. 10–1). The median nerve provides sensibility to the thumb and the volar aspects of the index finger, long finger, and half of the ring finger. The ulnar nerve provides sensibility to the small finger, the ulnar aspect of the ring finger, and to the ulnar side of the dorsum of the hand. The radial nerve provides sensibility to the radial border of the dorsum of the hand and the dorsum of the digits. The integrity of the motor function of the ulnar, median, and radial nerves easily can be tested as follows:

- Ulnar nerve motor function is ascertained by testing resisted abduction of the fingers while palpating over the first dorsal interosseous muscle in the first web space.
- Median nerve motor function in the opponens pollicis muscle is tested by asking the patient to touch the thumb and small finger together while the physician palpates the thenar musculature.
- The radial nerve innervates no intrinsic muscles in the hand, but extrinsic radial innervation can be tested by active extension of the MCP joints or by active extension of the thumb metacarpal.

Phalen's maneuver, used to assess the susceptibility of the median nerve to compression at the carpal tunnel, is performed by holding the wrist in maximal flexion. The appearance of paresthesias in the long and index fingers within 30 seconds is a positive test and may indicate carpal tunnel syndrome. *Tinel's sign* is elicited by gently tapping over the median nerve at the level of the palmar flexion crease. Paresthesias radiating to the index and long fingers constitute a positive test and may indicate carpal tunnel syndrome.

Circulation to the hand is assessed by observing the warmth and color of the fingertips, as well as by assessing capillary refill in the fingertips. Radial and ulnar arterial pulses should be palpated, but

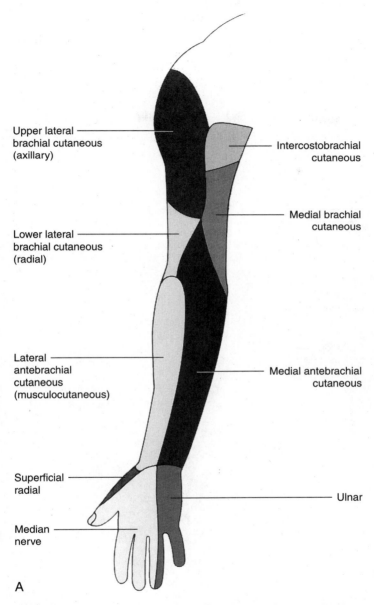

Upper lateral brachial cutaneous (axillary)

Intercostobrachial cutaneous

Medial brachial cutaneous

Lower lateral brachial cutaneous (radial)

Lateral antebrachial cutaneous (musculocutaneous)

Medial antebrachial cutaneous

Superficial radial

Ulnar

Median nerve

A

Figure 10–1 ◻ Anterior and posterior views of the upper limb, illustrating the peripheral nerve distribution for sensory innervation of the skin. (From Jenkins DB: Hollinshead's Functional Anatomy of the Limbs and Back, 6th ed. Philadelphia, WB Saunders, 1991, p 109.)

Continued on following page

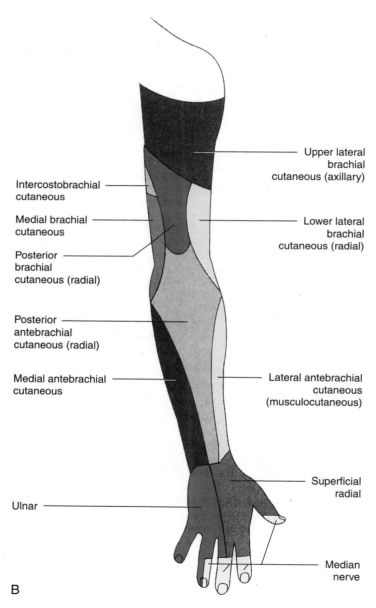

Upper lateral brachial cutaneous (axillary)

Intercostobrachial cutaneous

Medial brachial cutaneous

Posterior brachial cutaneous (radial)

Lower lateral brachial cutaneous (radial)

Posterior antebrachial cutaneous (radial)

Medial antebrachial cutaneous

Lateral antebrachial cutaneous (musculocutaneous)

Superficial radial

Ulnar

Median nerve

B

Figure 10–1 □ Continued

a palpable pulse does not always indicate good arterial inflow to the digits. *Allen's test* is performed to assess the relative contributions of the radial and ulnar arteries to digital blood flow. The patient is asked to make a tight fist; then the examiner compresses the radial and ulnar arteries with his fingers. The patient opens the hand and the examiner releases pressure on one of the arteries while observing the rapidity of capillary refill of the digit. The test is repeated, checking capillary fill from the other artery. Although capillary refill to the fingers should be present from either artery, the ulnar artery is usually the dominant circulation.

Further Orders

Radiographs of the hand should be obtained to exclude any bone pathology such as fracture, dislocation, or tumor of bone. The standard radiographic series includes AP, oblique, and lateral views of the hand. If the pathology involves a single finger, AP, oblique, and lateral views of that finger should be obtained. If infection is suspected, a CBC and ESR should be obtained.

■ MANAGEMENT

In the absence of infection, definitive management of atraumatic pain or numbness in the hand is not urgent. In cases of suspected infection, orthopaedic consultation should be obtained immediately, since prompt decompression and debridement of the infected area, in addition to appropriate antibiotic therapy, is necessary to prevent long-term disability. Although the hand can be immobilized for short periods, it is wise not to immobilize the hand unless absolutely necessary to stabilize unstable fractures. Most atraumatic disorders of the hand are treated with supportive management, including gentle range of motion exercises, edema control, NSAIDs, and occasional brief immobilization.

The initial management of suspected carpal tunnel syndrome generally consists of NSAIDs and a "cock-up" splint for the wrist, usually to be worn by the patient at night. Modification of activities that exacerbate the symptoms are also important; this may include work restrictions or modification of the workplace, particularly in the case of a patient who operates a keyboard or does other fine motor activity. Injection of corticosteroids into the carpal tunnel and performance of nerve conduction studies are generally reserved for patients whose symptoms do not resolve with the initial treatment modalities. Generally it is best to refer these patients to an orthopaedist for a more detailed evaluation and treatment.

Basilar arthritis of the thumb, a common condition seen most frequently in middle-aged women, is characterized by pain at the base of the thumb, especially with pinch, and by degenerative changes and subluxation on radiographs. Initial management consists of administration of NSAIDs and support of the thumb in a soft or rigid thumb spica splint. These patients should probably be referred to an orthopaedist, as treatment with injections or interposition arthroplasty frequently completely relieves pain and restores normal functioning of the thumb.

Pyogenic flexor tenosynovitis, or infection of a flexor tendon sheath, classically is manifested by a flexed, enlarged, sausagelike digit that is exquisitely tender on its palmar aspect and painful with passive extension. Recent minor penetrating trauma is the usual cause, and *Staphylococcus aureus* is typically the infecting organism. On rare occasions the infection may be successfully treated with antibiotics alone, but in most instances, surgical irrigation and drainage are required to cure the infection and return normal functioning to the digit.

Patients bitten by animals usually give reliable histories, but patients who sustain human bites are often reluctant to reveal the true cause of their injury. Any wound over a knuckle should be considered a human bite and treated as such until it can be proven otherwise. Bite wounds should *never* be closed primarily, and cultures should be obtained at the time of debridement. The patient should receive antibiotics and should be instructed to obtain follow-up within a few days of injury. Any bite injury that exposes extensor tendon should be presumed to have intraarticular involvement and should be irrigated and debrided surgically. The most common organisms causing infection after cat, dog, and human bites are sensitive to penicillin.

11

LOW BACK PAIN

Douglas R. Dirschl

Back pain is the most common patient complaint encountered by the practitioner of musculoskeletal medicine. If acute injuries are excluded, low back pain accounts for nearly one third of all outpatient clinic visits for musculoskeletal complaints. Patients with low back pain fall into two general categories. In the first category are patients with clear-cut physical signs that allow a precise determination of the nature and location of the lesion. In these patients a specific diagnosis can be made and curative treatment usually can be recommended. In the second category, undoubtedly larger than the first, are patients without clear-cut abnormalities on clinical or radiographic evaluation. Diagnosis in this group of patients cannot be made with certainty, and treatment is empiric. For lack of a more accurate term, the patients in this group are referred to as having *mechanical low back pain*.

Low back pain commonly radiates to the buttock or posterior thigh. When back pain radiates in this pattern and when the pattern of radiation is reproduced in a straight leg raise test, it is generally referred to as sciatica. Although still a manifestation of low back pain and not nerve root impingement, sciatica is a much more disturbing symptom to patients than is pain in the lower back. Careful education of patients as to the source of their back pain and reassurance that paralysis will not result are important in the management of these patients.

■ PHONE CALL

Questions

1. **How long has the pain been present?**

   The sudden onset of severe low back pain generally is related to an acute strain but may also represent a herniated disk or an infection. Chronic low back pain is usually mechanical in origin and rarely is associated with significant nerve root impingement.

2. **Does the pain radiate to the toes?**

   Radiation of the pain to the toes, especially if the pattern of radiation corresponds to the sensory distribution of a single lumbosacral nerve root, may indicate nerve root impingement from herniated nucleus pulposus.

3. **Does the patient complain of any numbness or weakness in the leg?**

   Many patients with low back pain will claim their leg "gives out" because of pain. Few, however, give a history suggestive of true muscular weakness in the leg or foot. Weakness in the foot or leg may be a sign of advanced nerve root impingement or even of compression of the cauda equina.

4. **Has the patient noted any changes in bowel or bladder sensibility?**

   Loss of normal bowel or bladder sensibility may indicate the patient is suffering from compression of the cauda equina within the lumbosacral vertebral canal, a serious condition. This often is noted by the patient as spotting of urine in the underwear. (The physician must remember, however, that the most common cause of spotting of urine, especially in females, is a urinary tract infection.)

Orders

None.

Inform RN

"I will arrive at the bedside/emergency department in 30 minutes." Although mechanical low back pain is common, radicular back pain, due to compression of a nerve root, and cauda equina syndrome, due to compression of the entire thecal sac and its contents, are much more serious conditions. Therefore it is prudent to evaluate patients with low back pain promptly.

■ ELEVATOR THOUGHTS

- Congenital abnormalities
  - Hemivertebra
  - Spina bifida
- Deformities
  - Scoliosis
  - Kyphosis
  - Hyperlordosis
- Infections of bone
  - Pyogenic infection of the spine
  - Tuberculosis of the spine
- Arthritis/arthrosis
  - Spondylosis (degenerative disk disease)
  - Rheumatoid arthritis
  - Osteoarthrosis
  - Ankylosing spondylitis

- Osteochondritis
    Scheuermann's disease
- Mechanical derangement
    Herniated intervertebral disk
    Spondylolysis
    Spondylolisthesis
    Spinal stenosis
    Cauda equina syndrome
- Tumors
    Osteoid osteoma
    Hemangioma
    Metastatic disease
- Chronic mechanical low back pain

■ BEDSIDE

Vital Signs

Vital signs generally are not necessary in the evaluation of atraumatic low back pain. If, however, infection is suspected, a full set of vital signs should be obtained.

Selective History

What is the specific location of the pain? Where does the pain radiate? What makes the pain better or worse?

Great effort should be made to ascertain the specific location of the pain, the pattern of any radiation, the time course of the pain, and the presence of any alleviating or exacerbating activities or positions. Particular attention should be paid to whether the pain occurs in the back, in the buttock, in the posterior thigh, in the leg, or in the foot. Most patients with low back pain are more comfortable standing or lying flat (positions in which the spine is in extension) than sitting (a position in which the spine is in flexion). The exception to this general rule is that patients with spinal stenosis are more comfortable when the spine is in flexion than in extension; this is because the spinal canal is larger when the spine is flexed, allowing more space for the thecal sac and its contents. Pain that is worse at night is common for nearly all back strains; however, pain that occurs only at night should prompt consideration of osteoid osteoma, a benign tumor of bone occasionally seen in the second and third decades of life.

Does the patient have any symptoms classic for herniated nucleus pulposus or cauda equina syndrome?

Patients should be questioned about any changes in bowel or bladder sensation; loss of or alterations in this sensation could be an indication of impending cauda equina syndrome. Numbness or weakness in a single nerve root distribution may be a sign of nerve root compression, whereas generalized bilateral weakness and progressive difficulty walking may be signs of impending cauda equina syndrome. The patient also should be asked if the pain first occurred with lifting or another activity that might have caused injury.

Does the patient have a previous history of low back pain or spinal conditions?

Prior infections of the spine, prior spinal surgeries, and a history of congenital abnormalities of the vertebrae may all be potential causes for low back pain. The physician should keep in mind that most adults who have had one episode of low back pain are likely to have another at some time in their lives. Although most of these patients with recurrent symptoms simply will have another low back strain, the physician should perform a complete physical evaluation to exclude other causes for the pain.

Selective Physical Examination

Inspection

With patient standing and disrobed, except for underwear, the physician should examine the bone contours and alignment of the spine, looking particularly for hyperlordosis, kyphosis, or scoliosis. Having the patient bend forward is a more sensitive way to identify scoliosis, since the rotational deformity of the scoliotic curve will become readily apparent (as a rib hump) with the patient bending forward. The color and texture of the skin should be assessed; a small patch of hair just above the sacrum may be indicative of an occult spina bifida. Finally, the patient's skin should be inspected for any scars or sinuses that might indicate an old injury, prior surgical procedures, or ongoing chronic infection.

Palpation

The back should be palpated for any specific sites of tenderness. Special attention should be paid to whether tenderness is directly over the spinous processes (in the midline) or over the paraspinous muscles (paramedian). Tenderness over the sciatic nerve as it emerges from beneath the gluteus maximus in the buttock can be indicative of nerve root irritation or inflammation.

Movements

The physician should instruct the patient to bend forward, lean backward, and bend to each side and should observe the actual range of motion and the patient's response to these movements. Marked muscle spasm and difficulty with these movements may indicate an acute inflammatory process, whereas excessive facial grimacing by the patient may be indicative of a psychosomatic component to the pain. Patients with inflammatory conditions will exhibit spinal movements that are limited by pain. Patients with spondylosis will have limited movements without pain, and patients with severe ankylosing spondylitis may have no movement of the spine whatsoever.

Neurologic Examination of the Lower Limbs

The physician should perform a careful and detailed motor and sensibility examination of both lower extremities. The examination should be focused on eliciting any decreased sensibility or weakness referable to a particular nerve root level. For example, the S1 nerve root supplies sensibility to the lateral border and sole of the foot, supplies power to the extensor hallucis longus muscle, and is the primary component of the Achilles reflex. Therefore, all three of these areas should be tested in assessing the S1 nerve root. The motor, sensory, and reflex components for the lumbosacral nerve roots are summarized in Table 11–1.

Finally, the physician should perform special tests to assess for nerve root irritation that may be indicative of herniated nucleus pulposus. With the patient supine, one should gently lift each lower limb in turn while holding the knee straight. Marked impairment of straight leg raising by pain in the back or thigh is indicative of mechanical low back pain or inflammation, whereas impairment of straight leg raising by pain in the leg or foot may be indicative of nerve root compression due to a herniated disk. The seated straight leg raise is performed with the patient seated on the end of the examination table with the legs over the sides. Each heel is raised in turn, extending the knee. The patient should be observed and asked about any symptoms on doing this. It is often helpful to distract the patient while doing this test, since it is important to ascertain whether the physical signs occur spontaneously or whether the patient elaborates when he believes his back is being tested.

Further Orders

If the onset of isolated low back pain is recent without any history of trauma and with normal neurologic findings on physical

Table 11–1 □ TESTING OF LUMBOSACRAL NERVE ROOTS

Root	Motor Innervation	Sensory Distribution	Reflex
L4	Tibialis anterior	Medial leg and medial foot	Quadriceps
L5	Extensor digitorum	Dorsum of foot	None
S1	Peroneus longus and brevis	Lateral and plantar foot	Achilles

examination, **plain radiographs are not immediately necessary.** Conservative treatment may be initiated and radiographs obtained in 4 to 6 weeks if the patient is having continued symptoms at that time. For all patients with a history of injury to the back or with physical findings indicating nerve root compression, scoliosis, or limited motion, radiographs should be obtained. A lumbosacral spine series, consisting of AP, lateral, and oblique views, is usually obtained. **An MRI scan should not be routinely obtained in patients with low back pain with normal neurologic findings.** An MRI scan is most useful as a preoperative planning study to aid the surgeon in determining the extent of surgical decompression, but the diagnosis of radiculopathy is primarily made on physical examination. An MRI only serves to confirm the clinical diagnosis and guide the surgical treatment of the condition.

■ MANAGEMENT

Most patients with low back pain (and even with radiculopathy) can be managed nonoperatively. Patients with acute or chronic low back pain should not be given large dosages of narcotic pain medications or antispasmodics; neither is particularly helpful for more than a few days, and both have great potential for abuse and addiction. Rather, patients should be given NSAIDs and noneuphoric antispasmodics, such as metalaxone (Skelaxin). Relative rest for the spine should be prescribed as well—complete bed rest is no longer recommended—and patients are advised to be up for personal care and household activities but to be recumbent when necessary to help relieve symptoms. The general concept is to avoid those activities that exacerbate the back pain but to avoid strict bed rest, which can result in severe muscle weakness and a slower overall recovery time.

It is important to counsel patients as to the nature of their low back pain. Although a definitive diagnosis cannot be made in all cases, it is important to inform the patient that his or her back pain is not due to cancer, a herniated disk, or some other condition that could lead to complete paralysis. Many patients with back pain fear paralysis, and reassurance that there is no risk of paralysis can be helpful to even the most severely afflicted patient.

Physical therapy with flexion or extension exercises or modalities such as ultrasound or phonophoresis can be helpful in acute cases of mechanical low back pain. In subacute or chronic cases, it is vital that the patient begin a daily program of regular exercise, abdominal strengthening, and hamstring stretching. The patient must be counseled that a lifetime program of these exercises will be necessary to help prevent further occurrences or worsening of low back pain.

Patients with hard neurologic findings of lumbosacral nerve root impairment or cauda equina syndrome should be referred immediately to an orthopaedist or a neurosurgeon for further evaluation and treatment.

Idiopathic scoliosis is not uncommon in females, is usually diagnosed in adolescence, and rarely is associated with pain. Any patient with scoliosis on examination should be referred to an orthopaedist for radiographic evaluation and discussion of treatment options. Most children with mild scoliosis are treated with observation, although children with more severe curvature of the spine may require bracing or surgical treatment.

Back pain in adolescents is rare, and although it most frequently is due to muscular strain and resolves spontaneously, the physician should be alert to the possibility of other sources of the pain. Radiographs should be obtained in all children and adolescents with low back pain. Possible causes include congenital abnormalities of the vertebrae, spondylolysis, spondylolisthesis, and hemangioma, and osteoid osteoma of the spine. All children with back pain and abnormalities on physical examination or radiographs should be referred to an orthopaedist for evaluation and treatment. In addition, children with low back pain and normal physical and radiographic findings whose symptoms do not resolve after 4 to 6 weeks of conservative management should also be referred to an orthopaedist for further evaluation.

Younger children may develop diskitis, a bacterial infection of the disk space between two vertebrae. These children usually will have severe back pain, will refuse to stand or walk because of pain, will have high fevers, and may appear septic. Radiographic findings may be minimal initially but may show slight widening of the disk space or formation of new bone surrounding the disk. An orthopaedic consultation should be obtained immediately in any child with suspected diskitis, as prompt initiation of appropriate antibiotics and, occasionally, surgical drainage are the cornerstones of successful treatment of this serious condition. Diskitis is discussed in greater detail in Chapter 37.

12

HIP PAIN

Douglas R. Dirschl

The wide range of pathologic conditions occurring around the hip constitute some of the most frequent and most fascinating problems in musculoskeletal medicine. In the child, hip disorders can result in abnormal development of the acetabulum, leading to functional limitations and pain at a very young age. In the adult, hip disorders can cause prolonged suffering and serious functional limitation. Physical evaluation of the hip is not particularly difficult but requires some experience. Time spent learning to examine the hip correctly usually will be well rewarded with an enhanced ability to easily and accurately diagnose hip disorders.

■ PHONE CALL

Questions

1. **How old is the patient?**

   Many serious hip disorders occur in childhood, often during a particular age range. This is so true with some disorders of the hip that the age of the patient at the onset of symptoms can afford some indication of the likely cause of hip pain, as shown in Table 12–1.

2. **How long has the pain been present?**

   The sudden onset of severe pain may indicate acute infection, acute slipped capital femoral epiphysis, sudden collapse of the femoral head associated with avascular necrosis, or fracture.

3. **What is the precise location of the pain (buttock, groin, lateral hip)?**

   Low back pain frequently radiates to the buttock, whereas pain from the hip joint usually is felt in the groin area. Pain over the lateral hip usually originates in the region of the greater trochanter or hip abductor muscles.

4. **Did the patient fall or sustain some other injury?**

   For a discussion of the evaluation and management of hip pain associated with trauma, see Chapter 29.

5. **Is the patient febrile?**

   Although not all patients with hip pain and a fever have septic arthritis, the physician should suspect and rule out septic arthritis in every febrile patient with the sudden onset of hip pain.

Table 12–1 □ **USUAL AGE AT DIAGNOSIS OF COMMON HIP DISORDERS**

Age (y)	Disease
0 to 2	Development dislocation
2 to 5	Transient synovitis, septic arthritis
5 to 10	Perthes' disease, transient synovitis
10 to 20	Slipped capital femoral epiphysis
20 to 50	Osteoarthritis (due to prior injury or disease)
50 to 100	Osteoarthritis (primary)

Orders

None.

Inform RN

"I will arrive at the bedside/emergency department in 15 to 30 minutes." Although hip pain without a history of trauma is rarely a true emergency, the possibility that the patient may have septic arthritis of the hip should prompt immediate evaluation. Septic arthritis can irreversibly damage articular cartilage in less than 24 hours; therefore patients with hip pain should be assessed promptly to rule out infection.

■ ELEVATOR THOUGHTS

- Congenital deformities
    Developmental dislocation of the hip
    Proximal femoral focal deficiency
    Coxa magna
    Coxa vara
- Arthritis/arthrosis
    Transient synovitis of children
    Pyogenic arthritis
    Tuberculous arthritis
    Rheumatoid arthritis
    Osteoarthrosis
- Osteochondritis
    Legg-Calvé-Perthes disease
- Physeal disorders
    Slipped capital femoral epiphysis
- Vascular disorders
    Avascular necrosis of the femoral head
- Mechanical disorders
    Trochanteric bursitis
    Iliotibial band syndrome

■ BEDSIDE

Vital Signs

Vital signs should be taken in all patients with hip pain. An elevated temperature and heart rate may be the earliest indications of septic arthritis, appearing before the symptoms and classic clinical signs of septic arthritis.

Selective History

What is the precise location of the pain?

It is extremely important to determine the precise location of the hip pain. Pain originating from the hip joint is perceived mainly in the groin and in the front or inner side of the thigh. Hip pain may also be referred to the knee; in fact, in slipped capital femoral epiphysis, pain in the knee is often the child's only initial complaint. In contrast, pain referred from the spine or posterior pelvis is perceived mainly in the gluteal region and may radiate down the back or outer side of the thigh. Pain over the lateral aspect of the hip almost always is due to greater trochanteric bursitis or iliotibial band friction. Pain caused by disease in the hip area is made worse by walking, whereas gluteal pain, referred from the spine, is aggravated by activities such as stooping or lifting and is often eased by standing and walking erect.

Selective Physical Examination

Inspection

With the patient disrobed, except for underwear, and lying supine, the pelvis should be inspected for bone and soft tissue contours. A tilted pelvis may be postural, or it may be indicative of a leg length discrepancy (Fig. 12–1). A patient with acute inflammation of the hip joint (transient synovitis or septic arthritis) will adopt a position of flexion of the hip when lying supine and will strongly resist any attempts to extend the affected hip. The color and texture of the skin should be assessed: erythema or localized swelling may indicate infection; scars may indicate old injuries or prior surgeries; and sinuses may indicate ongoing chronic infection.

Palpation

The skin over the hip region should be palpated for temperature, as septic arthritis initially may present only with local warmth. Bone prominences, as well as soft tissue regions, should be palpated for specific sites of tenderness, especially over the greater trochanter, the anterior hip joint capsule, and the iliac crest.

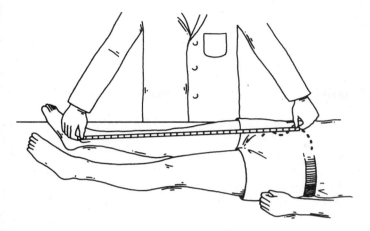

Figure 12–1 □ Pelvic tilt may produce the appearance of a leg length discrepancy. To determine true leg length, measure from the anterior superior iliac spine to the medial malleolus. (From Birnbaum JS: The Musculoskeletal Manual, 2nd ed. Philadelphia, WB Saunders, 1986, p 120.)

Movements

Passive range of motion of the hip should be assessed. Full extension of the hip is assessed by flexing the contralateral hip and observing that the other hip fully extends to lie flat on the bed or examining table (the *Thomas test*) (Fig. 12–2). Rotation of the hip generally is tested with the patient supine and the hip and knee flexed 90 degrees. Abduction of the hip is tested by stabilizing the pelvis while sliding the hip along the bed into abduction. Severe pain with extension of the hip or rigidly maintaining the hip in a flexed position can be signs of septic arthritis. Loss of internal rotation of the hip in a child may be the only sign of a slipped capital femoral epiphysis, whereas loss of rotation in the adult generally is due to osteoarthritis.

Special Tests

Greater trochanteric bursitis or tendinitis can be identified by locating tenderness directly over the greater trochanter and can be confirmed by reproducing the patient's pain with resisted abduction of the hip. This test is performed most easily by having the patient lie on the unaffected side and then asking the patient to raise the affected leg up into the air from that position.

The *Ober test* is performed with the patient lying on his or her side. The physician holds the patient's upward leg and extends the hip while flexing the knee. This test assesses tightness in the rectus

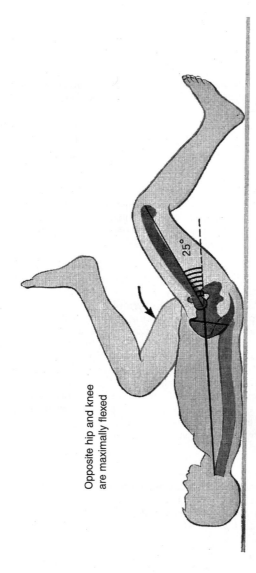

Opposite hip and knee
are maximally flexed

25°

Lumbar spine flattens   Note flexion contracture of hip

Figure 12–2 □ The Thomas test for hip flexion contracture (see text for description). Note that flexion of the contralateral hip flattens the lumbar spine and makes the hip flexion contracture apparent. (From Wiesel SW, Delahay JN: Essentials of Orthopaedic Surgery, 2nd ed. Philadelphia, WB Saunders, 1997, p 40.)

femoris portion of the quadriceps muscle, as well as in the iliotibial band.

Examination for Postural Stability

The *Trendelenburg test* is performed by having the patient alternately stand on one foot and then the other while the examiner palpates both iliac crests. In a Trendelenburg test positive for instability the contralateral pelvis drops in single limb stance or the patient leans markedly to the ipsilateral side to retain balance and keep a level pelvis (Fig. 12–3).

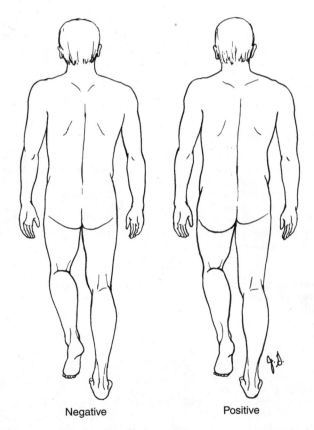

Negative   Positive

Figure 12–3 □ Trendelenburg test, measuring abductor strength. A positive test is associated with a sagging of the pelvis on the side opposite the weakness. In this figure the right side is affected. (From Borenstein DG, Wiesel SW, Boden SD: Low Back Pain: Medical Diagnosis and Comprehensive Management, 2nd ed. Philadelphia, WB Saunders, 1995, p 81.)

Further Orders

AP and lateral radiographs of the hip generally should be obtained in all patients with the initial onset of hip pain. In most situations a cross-table lateral of the hip is preferred; however, if slipped capital femoral epiphysis is suspected, a frog-leg lateral generally is preferred, as this allows better assessment of the position of the femoral head relative to the neck in this condition. If septic arthritis is suspected, a CBC, ESR, and blood cultures should be obtained, and aspiration of the affected hip under fluoroscopic guidance should be considered.

If avascular necrosis of the femoral head is suspected or confirmed on plain radiographic examination of the hip, an MRI scan of both hips may be indicated. The MRI scan will indicate the extent of the avascular region in the involved femoral head, as well as the presence of disease in the contralateral femoral head. This information is important in determining the most appropriate treatment for the patient, as well as for counseling the patient as to the likely outcome of treatment.

■ MANAGEMENT

Patients with suspected septic arthritis of the hip should be referred immediately to an orthopaedic surgeon for aspiration of the hip and for consideration of operative incision and drainage. Irreversible damage to articular cartilage has been noted in as few as 24 hours after the onset of septic arthritis, so prompt recognition and treatment are imperative.

Any child with clinical or radiographic evidence of a hip problem, such as developmental dysplasia, Perthes' disease, or slipped capital femoral epiphysis, should be kept non-weight-bearing on the affected limb and referred immediately to an orthopaedist.

Nonoperative management of osteoarthritis of the hip consists of weight loss, NSAIDs, and use of a cane if necessary to unweight the affected joint. Weight loss is emphasized because in single limb stance, joint reaction forces across the hip joint are three to four times body weight. Thus a 10 lb (4.5 kg) weight reduction results in a 30 to 40 lb (13.5 to 18 kg) decrease in force across the hip joint with every step. For biomechanical reasons a cane should be carried in the hand opposite the affected hip to most effectively unweight the painful joint.

Patients with greater trochanteric bursitis should be managed with NSAIDs and strengthening exercises for the abductor muscles on the affected side. Physical therapy is often helpful, and modalities such as ultrasound and phonophoresis, as applied by a physical therapist, can help greatly in alleviating the symptoms. Injection of the greater trochanteric area can be quite helpful in patients who do not respond to 4 to 6 weeks of medications and strengthening. Most frequently, bupivacaine and a corticosteroid are injected, the injection being 10 to 12 ml to ensure the entire area is infiltrated with medication.

Patients with avascular necrosis of the femoral head should be referred to an orthopaedist for further evaluation and management. Although not indicated in all patients, early surgical intervention in selected patients can relieve pain and may improve function, retard disease progression, and perhaps promote revascularization of the femoral head.

13

KNEE PAIN

Douglas R. Dirschl

Pain in or around the knee is one of the most common musculoskeletal complaints in all age groups. Children frequently experience "growing pains" around the knee. Knee pain in adults usually is due to an inflammatory condition or internal derangement. In the elderly, knee pain usually is due to osteoarthrosis. The knee is, in fact, a region where nearly every type of musculoskeletal disorder is commonly represented: developmental, inflammatory, infectious, mechanical, and degenerative.

The physician must not forget that hip pain commonly is referred to the knee. Thus the physician must be certain to examine the hip region in any patient, especially a child, who complains of knee pain. Not infrequently, a child with a slipped capital femoral epiphysis will present with a limp and knee pain in the absence of pain in the hip.

The knee depends for its stability on its four main ligaments and upon the quadriceps mechanism. Any pathologic condition that causes an imbalance in these structures can lead to knee pain and mechanical difficulties. The importance of the quadriceps mechanism in enhancing knee stability cannot be overemphasized; a powerful quadriceps mechanism can maintain stability of the knee despite laxity of the cruciate ligaments. In contrast, weakness or pain in the quadriceps will result in a limp and "giving way" of the knee, regardless of the integrity of the knee ligaments.

The knee particularly also is prone to every kind of arthritis. Moreover, it is a joint most commonly affected by osteochondritis dissecans and intraarticular loose body formation. The region about the child's knee is the site of the greatest longitudinal bone growth in the lower limb. Partly for this reason the portions of the femur and tibia near the knee are the most common sites of growing pains, osteomyelitis, and primary malignant bone tumors.

■ PHONE CALL

Questions

1. How old is the patient?

The age of the patient can give clues as to the likely cause of the knee pain. Knee pain in children usually is related to rapid growth or infection. Knee pain in young adults generally is related to mechanical derangement. In the elderly, knee pain usually is due to osteoarthrosis.

2. **How long have the symptoms been present?**
   The sudden onset of severe knee pain generally indicates an infection, acute mechanical derangement, loose body, or a flare-up of arthritis pain. In contrast, indolent or chronic knee pain generally is due to overuse or a degenerative condition.
3. **Does the pain radiate to any other areas?**
   Although it is not common for knee pain to radiate to other regions, hip pain commonly radiates to the knee. Complaints of knee pain radiating to the feet should prompt the physician to investigate sources for the pain other than the knee, such as the lower back or vascular or neurologic systems.
4. **Is the patient febrile?**
   Although not all patients with knee pain and a fever have septic arthritis, the physician should be certain to rule out septic arthritis in all febrile patients with knee pain.
5. **Is the patient able to bear weight on the leg?**
   As a general rule, patients with septic arthritis, osteomyelitis, major ligament disruption, or major fractures cannot bear weight on the affected knee. Although the patient's ability to bear weight on the painful knee may be an indication the disorder is not serious, the physician should perform a complete evaluation in all patients with knee pain.
6. **Has the patient sustained any recent injury to the knee?**
   For a discussion of the evaluation and management of knee pain associated with trauma, see Chapter 30.

Orders

None.

Inform RN

"I will arrive at the bedside/emergency department in 15 to 30 minutes." Although knee pain in the absence of trauma is unlikely to require urgent treatment, the possibility of septic arthritis or osteomyelitis mandates that the patient be seen promptly.

■ ELEVATOR THOUGHTS

Disorders of the Distal Femur and Proximal Tibia
- Infections
    Acute osteomyelitis
    Chronic osteomyelitis
    Nonpyogenic osteomyelitis
- Tumors
    Benign tumors of bone
    Malignant tumors of bone

- Miscellaneous disorders
    Apophysitis of the tibial tubercle (Osgood-Schlatter disease)

Articular Disorders of the Knee
- Arthritis / arthrosis
    Pyogenic arthritis
    Tuberculous arthritis
    Rheumatoid arthritis
    Osteoarthrosis
    Hemophilic arthritis
- Mechanical disorders
    Tears of the menisci
    Cysts of the menisci
    Discoid lateral meniscus
    Osteochondritis dissecans
    Intraarticular loose bodies
    Tear of the anterior or posterior cruciate ligaments
    Patellofemoral disorders
- Recurrent subluxator or dislocation of the patella
- Patellofemoral malalignment
- Chondromalacia patellae

Extraarticular Disorders of the Knee Region
- Prepatellar bursitis
- Semimembranosus bursitis
- Popliteal cyst
- Arthrofibrosis (frozen knee)

■ BEDSIDE

Vital Signs

Although most nontraumatic disorders of the knee will not cause any change in vital signs, the possibility of infection makes it necessary to obtain vital signs, particularly temperature, on all patients with the acute, atraumatic onset of pain and swelling in the knee.

Selective History

What was the mechanism of injury to the knee?

Knowledge of an injury is of particular importance in the diagnosis of disorders of the knee. In the case of a torn meniscus, for example, knowledge of a twisting injury may be the most important factor in making the diagnosis.

Does the patient have a history of knee pain or injury?

When there has been a previous injury to the knee, the precise mechanism of the injury and subsequent treatments should be ascertained. Questions should be asked regarding the ability to bear weight immediately after injury, the length of time before swelling became apparent, and the patient's ability to extend and flex the knee fully.

Does the patient experience locking or catching of the knee?

Although careful questioning is important in making the correct diagnosis of knee disorders, the physician should be cautious in accepting the patient's complaint of locking at face value. Many patients will complain of locking when the knee is stiff and painful or when it causes momentary flashes of pain on movement. True locking of the knee from a torn meniscus means that the knee cannot be straightened fully, although it usually can be flexed freely. With true locking of the knee due to entrapment of an intraarticular loose body the knee is truly stuck—it will neither flex nor extend.

Does the patient experience giving way of the knee?

As with locking, "giving way" is a common patient complaint that must not always be taken at face value. True giving way of the knee due to a deficient anterior cruciate ligament is painless; pain may occur later, but the giving way is experienced before the pain is. Pain inhibition of the quadriceps muscle can give the patient the sense the knee is giving way; in this case, however, the patient will experience the pain first, followed by the knee's giving way because of release of the quadriceps from pain inhibition, a normal protective response in striated muscle.

Selective Physical Examination

Inspection

The patient should be disrobed from the thighs downward. It is vital to have both lower extremities exposed to provide immediate comparison between the painful knee and the asymptomatic knee. With the patient supine and the knees fully extended, the examiner should look carefully at the bone and soft tissue contours and alignment of both knees. The examiner should pay particular attention to whether the symptomatic knee lies in full extension and to whether there is peripatellar swelling that might indicate a knee effusion. Prepatellar swelling also is easily identified and may indicate prepatellar bursitis. Erythema may indicate infection or an inflammatory condition. The heels should then be gently lifted and the knees compared to see if one or both knees hyperextend. Hyperextension on the symptomatic side but not on the other side may indicate a cruciate ligament injury. Both knees should then be flexed approximately 90 degrees with the feet resting on the examining table. Have the patient relax and look at the knees from the sides. A less prominent tibial tuberosity on the normal side (the posterior sag sign) indicates a posterior cruciate ligament injury. If one places a straight edge, such as an index card, on the tibial tuberosity on the normal knee, there will be a triangular clear space between the straight edge and the distal femur. In a patient with a positive posterior sag sign, however, the index card will contact the distal femur.

Palpation

The knees, once again extended, should be palpated carefully for any areas of tenderness and for a joint effusion. Effusion most easily is tested for by placing the thumb of one hand on the anterior surface of the patella while the thumb and the index finger of the other hand palpate the medial and lateral suprapatellar pouches. Alternate pressure and relaxation of the thumb on the patella will, if an effusion is present, elicit a fluid wave that can be felt in the palpating fingers. Tenderness directly over the patella may indicate an inflammatory condition, osteomyelitis, or prepatellar bursitis. Tenderness at the superior or inferior poles of the patella may indicate inflammation of the tendon insertion at that site. The knees are then flexed and further palpated for bone tenderness. Tenderness over the tibial tuberosity may indicate Osgood-Schlatter disease, whereas tenderness over the proximal medial tibia at the insertion of the semimembranosus muscle may indicate semimembranosus bursitis. Tenderness over the femoral origin of the medial collateral ligament may indicate a medial collateral ligament tear, whereas tenderness over the medial or lateral joint lines may indicate a meniscal tear. Tenderness, warmth, and erythema over the proximal tibia are characteristic of proximal tibial osteomyelitis.

Girth of each thigh should be measured with the knee fully extended and the patient relaxed. Atrophy of the thigh musculature on the injured side will be signaled by a smaller thigh girth. Quadriceps atrophy can be indicative of disuse of the knee because of pain or injury.

Movements

The active and passive range of motion of each knee should be carefully assessed, keeping in mind that 0 degree represents full extension and 135 degrees represents maximal knee flexion. Passive extension of 0 degree with active extension only to 45 degrees indicates weakness in the quadriceps mechanism and is referred to as an *extensor lag*. If, however, passive knee extension is not 0 degree, the patient is said to exhibit a *flexion contracture*. A patient with a septic knee will hold the knee in midflexion and will strongly resist either flexion or extension from that position.

Stability

Integrity of the medial and lateral collateral ligaments is tested with the knee in full extension and in 20 degrees of flexion. With the knee held in these positions, varus and valgus forces are exerted on the knee, and the patient's pain response and the degree of opening of the joint lines are recorded. These responses are then compared to those of the other side. Pain on valgus stress with no laxity indicates a grade I tear of the medial collateral ligament; in contrast, pain and opening of the joint in excess of that on the contralateral side indicate a more severe tear of the medial collateral ligament.

The anterior cruciate ligament may be tested in a number of ways. The *anterior drawer test* is performed with the knee flexed 90 degrees and the foot resting on the examination table. The examiner stabilizes the patient's foot by sitting on it while grasping the proximal tibia with both hands. The examiner palpates for relaxation of the hamstrings, then pulls anteriorly on the proximal tibia. The amount of translation and the firmness of the endpoint are recorded. Greater translation and a softer endpoint than found on the contralateral side indicate an anterior cruciate ligament tear. The *Lachman test* is performed with the knee in 20 degrees of flexion. The examiner supports the lateral thigh with one hand while grasping the medial portion of the proximal tibia with the other. The examiner then pulls anteriorly with the hand holding the tibia and compares the excursion and firmness of the endpoint with that of the other knee. The *pivot shift test* is performed with the patient's knee in full extension: After axial loading, internal rotation, and valgus stresses are applied, the knee is slowly flexed. At approximately 30 degrees of flexion, a sudden shift in the lateral joint line will indicate a tear of the anterior cruciate ligament. If present, the shift should also be apparent on slowly extending the knee while performing the examination.

The integrity of the posterior cruciate ligament is tested most commonly by performing a *posterior drawer test* (the reverse of the anterior drawer test) or by observing a posterior sag sign on inspection of the flexed and relaxed knee.

Examination for a medial meniscal tear consists of searching for joint tenderness precisely at the joint line as well as performance of the McMurray test. The *McMurray test* is performed by fully flexing the knee and then flexing and extending the knee while rotating the tibia in internal and external rotation. A palpable or audible click at the joint line may indicate a meniscal tear: A displaced tag of the meniscal tear temporarily becomes impinged between the tibial and femoral articular surfaces. When the displaced meniscal fragment moves out of the impinged position, the click or pop is felt.

Further Orders

Radiographs of the knee are ordered in nearly all patients with knee pain. If the knee pain is acute or there is a knee effusion, a standard series of radiographs should be obtained. These consist of

AP, lateral, notch, and sunrise views. The notch view allows the physician to see the intercondylar notch of the distal femur and to identify any osteophytes and loose bodies in this region. The sunrise view, a tangential view of the patellofemoral joint, is used to assess patellofemoral arthritis as well as patellofemoral alignment in patients with recurrent patellar subluxation.

If the patient's knee pain occurs principally with weight bearing, as in osteoarthrosis, radiographs should be obtained with the patient standing. AP and lateral radiographs with the patient standing are obtained on 17-inch x-ray cassettes. Weight-bearing films are obtained to see the true alignment of the knee joint and the extent of joint space narrowing with the patient bearing full weight. Long x-ray cassettes are used as they better show the overall varus or valgus alignment of the knee.

■ MANAGEMENT

Patients with suspected acute osteomyelitis or septic arthritis should be referred immediately to an orthopaedist for evaluation, aspiration of the bone or joint, and consideration for operative treatment.

Patients with suspected tears of the cruciate or collateral ligaments should be referred to an orthopaedist for definitive evaluation and treatment. The patient may be placed into a knee immobilizer for comfort; however, knee range of motion out of the brace should also be encouraged. Crutches may be used if ambulation is painful.

Patients with suspected tear of the medial or lateral meniscus may be treated nonoperatively, with NSAIDs, range of motion exercises, weight bearing as tolerated, and physical therapy. If the meniscus tear is displaceable, however, symptoms of locking will continue. These patients should be referred to an orthopaedist for evaluation and treatment.

Patients with inflammatory conditions about the knee, such as bursitis or a knee sprain, should be treated with NSAIDs, range of motion exercises, weight bearing as tolerated, and physical therapy.

Patients with osteoarthrosis of the knees should be informed of their diagnosis and of the slow, inexorable progression of the degenerative changes. They may be managed with NSAIDs or acetaminophen, weight loss, use of a cane, or occasionally with intraarticular corticosteroid injections. Patients with severe disease, severe limitation of ambulation because of knee pain, or worsening symptoms should be referred to an orthopaedist for evaluation and treatment.

Patients with osteochondritis dissecans of the knee or with osteochondral loose bodies on radiographs should be referred to an orthopaedist for evaluation and removal of the loose fragments.

Patients with insertional pain in the quadriceps at the superior border of the patella, in the patellar tendon at the distal pole of the patella, or at the insertion of the patellar tendon on the tibial tuberosity can all be treated similarly. Conservative treatment consists of an elastic bandage, NSAIDs, range of motion exercises of the knee, and the avoidance of activities that put severe stress on the knee and exacerbate symptoms. Physical therapy and the use of modalities such as ultrasound may also be considered. Failure to improve after 4 to 6 weeks of a conservative regimen is an indication for referral to an orthopaedist.

14

LEG PAIN

Douglas R. Dirschl

The leg is defined as the portion of the lower limb between the knee and the ankle; this encompasses the tibia and fibula, the muscles of the leg, and the veins, arteries, and nerves that traverse the leg in passing to the foot. Pain in the leg in the absence of trauma is an uncommon musculoskeletal complaint but one that can have a variety of causes. Overuse, infection, neurologic disorders, and tumors can all cause leg pain in the absence of trauma. A thorough history and careful physical examination is often all that is necessary to elicit the source of the patient's symptoms.

■ PHONE CALL

Questions

1. How long has the pain been present?

The sudden onset of severe leg pain may indicate infection, acute muscle tear, or fracture.

2. Is the pain related to activity?

Common causes for leg pain occurring only with activity are shin splints, vascular claudication, and exertional compartment syndrome.

3. Does the pain radiate to another location?

Leg pain rarely radiates to another location. Leg pain radiating to the feet should prompt the physician to search for a vascular or neurologic cause for the pain.

4. Is there swelling of the leg? If the leg is swollen, is the calf soft or taut? Does the patient have normal feeling in the toes?

Swelling of the leg is a nonspecific finding and may indicate peripheral edema, infection, tumor, hemorrhage, or deep venous thrombosis. A swollen, taut leg with loss of normal sensibility in the toes may indicate developing compartment syndrome. See Chapter 32 for a more detailed discussion of the evaluation and treatment of compartment syndrome.

Orders

None.

Inform RN

"I will arrive at the bedside/emergency department in 30 to 60 minutes." Although leg pain without antecedent trauma usually does not require urgent evaluation, the possibility of compartment syndrome or infection in the leg warrants prompt evaluation of these patients.

■ ELEVATOR THOUGHTS

- Overuse injuries
    - Stress fracture of the tibia
    - Shin splints
    - Rupture of the Achilles tendon
- Infections
    - Acute and chronic osteomyelitis
    - Nonpyogenic osteomyelitis
    - Soft tissue abscess
- Tumors
    - Benign and malignant tumors of bone
    - Benign and malignant tumors of soft tissue
- Circulatory disturbances
    - Intermittent claudication
    - Peripheral edema
    - Deep venous thrombosis
- Compartment syndrome
    - Acute compartment syndrome in the hemophiliac
    - Exertional compartment syndrome
- Neurologic disorders
    - Peripheral neuritis or neuropathy
    - Lumbar radiculopathy
    - Resolving peroneal nerve palsy

■ BEDSIDE

Vital Signs

In evaluation of the patient with leg pain without trauma, vital signs usually are not necessary. If, however, infection is suspected, the vital signs of the patient should be obtained.

Selective History

Does the patient have a history of back or leg problems?
The history of any previous disorders affecting the back or leg should be elicited. For example, a history of herniated nucleus pulposus may lead the physician to carefully evaluate whether the leg pain could be related to radiculopathy from scar tissue or

recurrent disc herniation. A history of previous peroneal nerve palsy might lead the physician to suspect that leg pain could be reinnervation pain as a part of the healing process of the peroneal nerve. A history of previous deep venous thrombosis of the leg may lead the physician to suspect that a recurrent deep venous thrombosis may be the source of the patient's symptoms.

What is the precise location of the pain?

The precise distribution of the pain should be carefully ascertained. Pain in the distribution of the peroneal nerve often is due to dysfunction of that nerve. Pain in the posteromedial tibia often is due to shin splints.

Is the pain present or worse only after activities?

Specific inquiries should be made as to the effect of standing and walking on the symptoms. Pain in the leg that occurs only after walking or running for a period of time may indicate claudication, exertional compartment syndrome, or stress fracture.

Selective Physical Examination

Inspection

It is essential that both limbs be exposed to above the knee for thorough examination of the leg. Initial inspection should examine soft tissue and bone contours and compare them with those of the contralateral limb. In particular, the examining physician should search for edema of the leg, any deformity or excrescence on the subcutaneous surface of the tibia, or an obvious local mass within the leg.

Palpation

The skin should be assessed for areas of local warmth, and the bone and soft tissue contours should be carefully palpated and compared to those of the other limb. Local tenderness should be sought and its precise location ascertained. Tenderness directly over the tibia in one location may indicate osteomyelitis, bone tumor, or stress fracture. Tenderness over the posteromedial border of the tibia generally indicates shin splints. Tenderness and reproduction of symptoms during palpation over the peroneal nerve generally indicates dysfunction or irritation of this nerve. A defect in the Achilles tendon near its insertion on the calcaneus indicates rupture of this structure.

Status of Peripheral Circulation

The feet should be examined for cyanosis when the leg is dependent. The absence of hair and the presence of chronic trophic skin changes may indicate vascular insufficiency. The dorsalis pedis and posterior tibialis pulses should be palpated, and capillary refill in the toes ascertained.

Compartment syndrome is a rare condition in which the pressure in the soft tissues of the leg is elevated to the extent that the vascular supply to the nerves and muscles in the leg is compromised. Compartment syndrome most often is the result of acute, massive trauma but may also occur transiently after athletic activity. Compartment syndrome is manifested by pain, compromised capillary refill to the toes, swelling of the leg, and paresthesias. Compartment syndrome is discussed in greater detail in Chapter 32.

Further Orders

Plain radiographs of the leg should be obtained if infection, stress fracture, bone tumor, or shin splints are suspected. AP and lateral radiographs that include both the knee and ankle joints should be obtained and carefully examined for bone changes. If a stress fracture of the tibia is suspected, oblique views may be the only views on which the fracture appears. If arterial insufficiency is suspected, arterial Doppler scans or segmental arterial pressures should be obtained. If deep venous thrombosis is suspected, venous Doppler scans of both lower extremities should be obtained. If peroneal nerve function is impaired, consideration could be given to obtaining nerve conduction studies.

■ MANAGEMENT

Chronic peripheral vascular insufficiency and peripheral edema due to heart failure are best managed according to principles of managing the causative condition. See textbooks of internal medicine.

Shin splints and stress fractures of the tibia are generally managed by modification of activities to reduce impact loading and symptoms, icing before and after physical activity, and administration of NSAIDs. If this treatment does not ameliorate symptoms in 4 to 6 weeks, referral to an orthopaedist should be considered.

Rupture of the Achilles tendon generally is managed by operative repair; however, nonoperative treatment can be successful and often is recommended in patients whose physical activities are not demanding. This condition is best managed by referral to an orthopaedist.

Suspected infection, abscess, or tumor should be managed by referral to an orthopaedist.

Exertional compartment syndrome can be treated conservatively with activity modifications and icing before and after athletic activities. If these measures fail to control symptoms, evaluation by an orthopaedist is indicated. Acute compartment syndrome or acute hemorrhage into the leg in a hemophiliac calls for immediate consultation with an orthopaedist.

Neuritis or other dysfunction of the peroneal nerve probably is managed best by referral to a neurologist or an orthopaedist.

15

ANKLE PAIN

Douglas R. Dirschl

The ankle is a common site for injury; sprains, tendinitis, and fractures occur commonly in all age groups. Ankle pain in the absence of injury is, however, rare. Although the ankle is spared somewhat from osteoarthrosis, inflammatory arthropathies are not uncommon. Most patients with atraumatic ankle pain can be successfully managed nonoperatively, but a careful history and physical examination will aid the physician in determining which patients require consultation with an orthopaedist.

■ PHONE CALL

Questions

1. **How long have the symptoms been present?**
   The sudden onset of severe ankle pain in the absence of trauma may indicate an infection, tendon rupture, or acute attack of inflammatory arthritis.
2. **Has the patient sustained an injury?**
   For a more detailed discussion of the evaluation and management of ankle pain following injury, see Chapter 33.
3. **Is the patient able to bear weight on the painful ankle?**
   As a general rule the patient who is able to walk on a painful ankle does not have a serious infection or inflammatory disorder.
4. **Is there warmth or erythema?**
   Although warmth and erythema are signs of acute infection, they are also present in acute tendinitis and inflammatory arthropathies.

Orders

None.

Inform RN

"I will arrive at the bedside/emergency department in 60 minutes." With the exception of septic arthritis, ankle pain in the absence of trauma rarely requires urgent management.

■ ELEVATOR THOUGHTS

- Arthritis / arthrosis
    Pyogenic arthritis
    Rheumatoid arthritis
    Osteoarthrosis
    Gouty arthritis
    Neuropathic arthropathy
- Posttraumatic mechanical derangements
    Recurrent subluxation
    Osteochondral loose bodies
    Formation of osseous spurs

■ BEDSIDE

Vital Signs

In general, vital signs are not necessary in the evaluation of ankle pain. If, however, infection is suspected, vital signs should be obtained.

Selective History

What is the precise location of the pain?

In nearly all cases, symptoms in the ankle can be explained by local disorders; only rarely is ankle pain referred from a distant location. The precise distribution and location of the pain should be ascertained, as well as the time of onset of symptoms.

Is the pain present or worse only with activities?

The effects of weight bearing and activity on the pain should also be ascertained. Inflammatory conditions usually are characterized by constant pain, whereas mechanical and degenerative conditions more often are characterized by pain with weight bearing or physical activity.

Does the patient have a history of ankle injury or ankle problems?

If the patient has had remote ankle trauma, the full details of the injury should be obtained. A history of rheumatoid arthritis or gout should be sought, since flare-ups of these conditions occur frequently and can be extremely painful.

Selective Physical Examination

Inspection

Both legs should be exposed from the knee distally to allow for examination and comparison with the contralateral asymptomatic side. The physician should note any swelling or erythema about the ankle, which might indicate injury, infection, or gout. Attention also should be paid to the bone contours as well as the presence of any scars or sinuses that might indicate previous injury, surgery, or chronic infection.

Palpation

The skin temperature should be assessed; warmth may be an indication of underlying inflammation or infection. The soft tissues and bones around the ankle should be palpated, with particular attention paid to the precise location of any tenderness. Tenderness over the medial or lateral malleolus may indicate an acute or old fracture. Tenderness over the anterior joint line may indicate arthritis. Tenderness over the lateral ankle ligaments may indicate an acute or old sprain. Global tenderness may indicate an inflammatory or infectious process. Tenderness localized to the joint line generally indicates an intraarticular disorder.

Movements

Active and passive range of motion of the ankle should be assessed. The neutral position of the ankle is defined as the ankle position that puts the sole of the foot at 90 degrees to the leg. Ankle dorsiflexion is motion into extension beyond neutral. Normal dorsiflexion is about 20 degrees. Ankle plantar flexion is normally about 30 to 35 degrees.

Stability

The integrity of the lateral ankle ligaments is assessed with the anterior drawer test. One hand is used to stabilize the anterior tibia in its distal one third while the contralateral hand grasps the calcaneus posteriorly. While anterior pressure is applied with the hand on the tibia, the calcaneus is forced forward and into internal rotation in the ankle mortise. Pain and greater translation than elicited in the contralateral ankle may be indicative of chronic ankle instability.

Further Orders

Radiographs of the ankle should be obtained in nearly all patients with ankle pain. An ankle series includes an AP, a lateral, and a mortise radiograph. These radiographs should be examined carefully for any signs of fracture, tumor, osteomyelitis, osteoarthritis, or osteochondral fragmentation of the medial or lateral corners of the talar dome. In cases of suspected infection, bone or MRI scans might also be helpful.

■ MANAGEMENT

With the exception of infection, nearly all atraumatic conditions of the ankle can be managed nonoperatively, and all are managed in a similar fashion: range of motion exercises; NSAIDs; wrapping or bracing for support; strengthening exercises for the peroneal, gastrosoleus, and anterior tibial muscles; and relative rest from activities that exacerbate symptoms. In most cases the patient should be counseled that the ankle is stable and safe for weight bearing but that only with time and careful treatment will the pain abate.

Patients with fractures, suspected infection, severe osteoarthritis, or osteochondral loose bodies should be referred to an orthopaedist for further evaluation and management.

Although acute gouty arthritis can be treated medically, aspiration of the ankle is required to make the diagnosis of gout and to rule out septic arthritis. Unless the physician is experienced in the aspiration of joints, orthopaedic consultation is recommended. Once the diagnosis of gout is confirmed, treatment of the acute crystalline arthropathy can be accomplished with either indomethacin or colchicine.

16

HEEL PAIN

Douglas R. Dirschl

Pain in or about the heel is one of the most common lower extremity complaints in patients with musculoskeletal disorders. Heel pain is a commonly used but somewhat nebulous term and may mean entirely different things to different patients. For the purpose of this chapter the heel refers to the area from the Achilles tendon insertion on the calcaneus to the proximal portion of the arch of the foot (Fig. 16–1).

■ PHONE CALL

Questions

1. **How old is the patient?**

   Knowing whether the patient is a child or an adult is helpful, as some conditions about the heel are much more common in children than in adults. For example, inflammation or apophysitis at the insertion of the Achilles tendon on the calcaneus (Sever's disease) and tarsal coalition can both cause heel pain in children but do not occur in adults.

2. **How long have the symptoms been present?**

   A sudden onset of severe heel pain may indicate a fracture or a tendon rupture, whereas the insidious onset of heel pain generally indicates a degenerative or overuse condition.

3. **Has the patient sustained an injury?**

   For a detailed discussion of heel pain associated with trauma, see Chapter 34.

4. **Is the pain present only with weight bearing or is it present at all times?**

   Pain with weight bearing generally is associated with overuse conditions, whereas constant pain is more common with acute inflammatory conditions, infection, or injuries.

5. **Has the patient experienced similar pain in the past?**

   A prior history of injury to or disorder in the heel should lead the physician to suspect the current symptoms may be caused by the same condition.

6. **What is the precise location of the pain?**

   The specific location of the pain can give great clues as to the likely diagnosis.

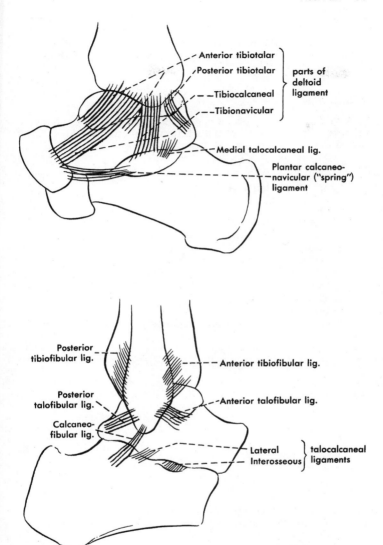

Figure 16–1 □ The heel refers to the area from the attachment of the Achilles tendon to the beginning of the arch of the foot. Ligaments of the heel region are shown. (From Jenkins DB: Hollinshead's Functional Anatomy of the Limbs and Back, 6th ed. Philadelphia, WB Saunders, 1991, p 312.)

Orders

No orders are necessary before the physician evaluates the patient. If, however, infection is suspected, a CBC and ESR should be obtained.

Inform RN

"I will arrive at the bedside/emergency department in 30 to 60 minutes." In the absence of acute trauma, pain in the heel need not be evaluated emergently.

■ ELEVATOR THOUGHTS

- Injuries
    - Rupture of the Achilles tendon
    - Stress fracture of the calcaneus
- Infections
    - Chronic and acute osteomyelitis
    - Soft tissue ulcerations and infections
- Overuse injuries
    - Achilles tendinitis
    - Retrocalcaneal bursitis
    - Haglund's disease ("pump bumps")
    - Plantar fasciitis
- Developmental conditions
    - Congenital clubfoot (talipes equinovarus)
    - Tarsal coalition
    - Sever's disease
- Neurologic disorders
    - Tarsal tunnel syndrome
    - Charcot's arthropathy

■ BEDSIDE

Vital Signs

Unless infection is strongly suspected, determination of vital signs is not required in the evaluation of nontraumatic heel pain.

Selective History

Is the patient diabetic?

Diabetes is a common disease in North America that often goes undiagnosed for many years. Patients with diabetes develop peripheral neuropathy, which most often affects the feet. This loss of the normal protective sensibility can lead to pressure ulcerations over many surfaces of the foot, including the plantar aspect of the heel. Humans rely on painful feedback to warn them of increased pressure on soft tissues. When pain is not present, as in the diabetic, ulcerations and soft tissue infections of the foot are common. On the other hand, neuropathic arthropathy (Charcot's arthropathy) can be painful, contrary to popular belief.

How long has the pain been present?

Acute onset of pain often indicates injury or infection, whereas the insidious onset of chronic pain usually indicates an overuse or degenerative condition.

Does the patient have a history of foot problems?

A history of childhood deformities of the foot (such as club-foot or congenital flatfoot) can be a vital clue as to the source of heel pain in the adult patient. Similarly, patients with a history of plantar fasciitis or Achilles tendinitis are likely to have a painful recurrence of these conditions.

What is the patient's occupation and normal activity level?

It is important to assess what stresses the patient's foot normally is subjected to. Stresses endured by the heel in the patient who spends the entire day walking on cement floors at work is much greater than those in the patient who spends his or her days seated at a desk.

What shoes does the patient normally wear?

In all patients with foot pain or deformity the physician should assess the patient's shoe wear and even examine the shoes themselves if possible; ill-fitting shoes or those that give poor support are common causes of heel and foot pain.

Selective Physical Examination

Inspection

It is essential for thorough examination of the heel or foot that socks or stockings be removed and that both legs be exposed to the knee. Both feet should be examined, and the painful foot compared to the asymptomatic one. The heels should be examined, with the patient both seated and standing, for swelling, symmetry, and deformity. Swelling in the area of the posterior heel, near the Achilles tendon insertion, may indicate Achilles tendinitis or retrocalcaneal bursitis. When viewed from behind, the standing patient's heels normally tilt slightly into valgus; when the patient raises up on his or her toes, the heels move into varus. Any alteration from this relationship or asymmetry from one heel to the other may indicate a disorder in the heel or subtalar joint complex. The skin of the heel should be inspected carefully for areas of erythema or ulceration.

Palpation

The heel should be carefully palpated for any areas of warmth or erythema, which may indicate deep infection. Each area of the heel should be carefully palpated with a single finger, searching for focal areas of fullness or tenderness. A defect in the Achilles tendon near its insertion into the calcaneus nearly always indicates an acute rupture of the Achilles tendon at its insertion. An intact Achilles tendon with tenderness directly over the tendon itself usually indicates Achilles tendinitis. Tenderness over the medial and lateral facets of the upper portion of the calcaneus (deep to the Achilles tendon) generally indicates retrocalcaneal bursitis or Haglund's disease. Tenderness directly overlying the posterior aspect of the calcaneus in a child suggests calcaneal apophysitis (Sever's disease). Tenderness over the plantar surface of the heel, especially directly at the origin of the plantar fascia, usually indicates plantar fasciitis. Tenderness over the medial portion of the calcaneus in the area just posterior to the medial malleolus may indicate posterior tibial tendinitis or tarsal tunnel syndrome.

Movements

The only movements that need be assessed in the heel are those of the subtalar joint complex. It is impossible to isolate the subtalar joint for motion testing, since in normal use the subtalar and midtarsal joints work together as a unit to permit inversion and eversion of the hindfoot. To test subtalar movements the physician supports the lower leg by gripping the ankle while lightly grasping the plantar surface of the calcaneus with the opposite hand. With the patient relaxed, the heel alternately is inverted and everted, and the range of motion is observed. The neutral position is considered to be that with the heel directly in line with the leg. The range of motion should be compared with that of the contralateral extremity. The normal range of motion is about 20 degrees of eversion and 15 degrees of inversion of the heel.

Special Tests

Tests for Tarsal Tunnel Syndrome.   Compression of the posterior tibial nerve behind the medial malleolus is referred to as tarsal tunnel syndrome (Fig. 16–2). This syndrome has varying clinical presentations. Two of the most common are pain in the plantar and medial aspects of the heel and numbness and tingling in some or all of the toes. The first branch of the posterior tibial nerve distal to the medial malleolus is the medial calcaneal branch, which supplies the skin over the medial side and the plantar surface of the heel. Decreased sensibility in the distribution of this nerve may indicate tarsal tunnel syndrome. In addition, gentle tapping over the posterior tibial nerve behind the medial malleolus may elicit dysesthesias in the distribution of the poste-

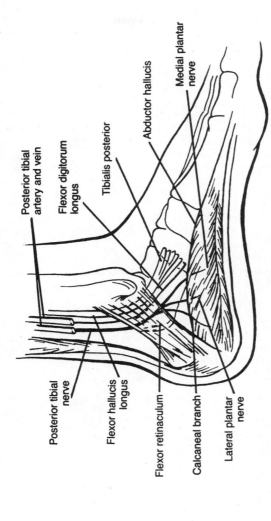

Figure 16–2 □ Tarsal tunnel syndrome is a result of compression of the posterior tibial nerve behind the medial malleolus. The figure indicates the relevant anatomic structures in the region. (From Gould JS: Operative Foot Surgery. Philadelphia, WB Saunders, 1994, p 188.)

Posterior tibial artery and vein

Flexor digitorum longus

Tibialis posterior

Abductor hallucis

Medial plantar nerve

Posterior tibial nerve

Flexor hallucis longus

Flexor retinaculum

Calcaneal branch

Lateral plantar nerve

rior tibial nerve. This finding (*Tinel's sign*) is also indicative of tarsal tunnel syndrome.

Tests for Posterior Tibial Tendinitis. Tenderness directly over the posterior tibial tendon, which lies directly posterior to the medial malleolus, may indicate posterior tibial tendinitis. Further testing can be performed by realizing that the posterior tibial tendon plantar flexes the ankle and inverts the foot. Resisted plantar flexion and inversion generally reproduce the pain in patients with posterior tibial tendinitis.

Tests for Plantar Fasciitis. The plantar fascia arises from the tubercle on the plantar surface of the calcaneus and extends the length of the foot, going beyond the metatarsophalangeal joints and inserting distally on the plantar aspect of the toes (Fig. 16–3). Given its anatomic location, combined dorsiflexion of the ankle and the toes puts maximal stretch on the plantar fascia. If this maneuver reproduces the patient's pain at the plantar aspect of the heel, a presumptive diagnosis of plantar fasciitis can be made.

Further Orders

If stress fracture, tarsal coalition, retrocalcaneal bursitis, or Achilles tendon rupture is suspected, plain radiographs of the foot may be helpful. Plain radiographs may show an Achilles tendon rupture if the rupture has occurred through the bone or previously calcified tendon. Stress fractures of the calcaneus also may be seen

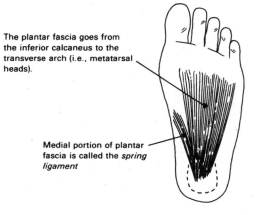

The plantar fascia goes from the inferior calcaneus to the transverse arch (i.e., metatarsal heads).

Medial portion of plantar fascia is called the *spring ligament*

Figure 16–3 □ The plantar fascia extends from the planar surface of the calcaneus to the plantar aspects of the toes. (From Birnbaum JS: The Musculoskeletal Manual, 2nd ed. Philadelphia, WB Saunders, 1986, p 231.)

on plain radiographs. An axial view of the heel (Harris heel view), however, often is necessary to evaluate the calcaneal tuberosity for stress fracture. The subtalar joint can be evaluated by plain radiographs of the foot (AP, oblique, and lateral views), but the subtalar joint complex is more clearly seen with special radiographic studies. Broden's view is helpful for viewing the posterior facet of the calcaneus, but it is not used commonly in clinical practice. Computed tomography (CT) is the most accepted means for evaluating the subtalar joint for arthritis or tarsal coalition. Radiographs of the foot are generally not helpful in patients with suspected plantar fasciitis. Heel spurs are seen on the lateral foot radiographs of approximately 50% of patients with plantar fasciitis and 50% of patients with no symptoms of heel pain. The presence of a heel spur on radiographs, then, is not helpful in generating the diagnosis of or dictating the management for plantar fasciitis.

■ MANAGEMENT

Rupture of the Achilles Tendon

Patients with rupture of the Achilles tendon should be referred to an orthopaedic consultant for evaluation and further management. Although ruptures of the Achilles tendon can be treated nonoperatively by placing the patient in a cast with the ankle in plantar flexion, the rate of rerupture is much higher with this treatment than with operative repair of the tendon. Therefore most orthopaedists recommend operative repair of ruptures of the Achilles tendon.

Achilles Tendinitis and Retrocalcaneal Bursitis

These conditions are treated, as are all overuse and inflammatory conditions, by the principles of rest, control of inflammation, and stretching. Patients with Achilles tendinitis or retrocalcaneal bursitis should be treated with NSAIDs, restriction of activities that worsen symptoms, ice prior to and following activities, and with a heel lift or other device to elevate the heel of the foot during weight bearing and thus remove some stress from the Achilles tendon region. Stretching of the Achilles tendon can relieve tightness and lessen the chance of further episodes of inflammation. Physical therapy can be helpful in patients who are not motivated or who cannot understand how to perform stretching exercises at home. Physical therapists can also apply treatments to the heel that may speed reduction of the inflammation and enhance the healing response. Injections of local anesthetics and corticosteroids into the retrocalcaneal bursa may be helpful in patients with retrocalcaneal bursitis but, in our experience, are rarely curative. Corticosteroids should never be injected within the substance of the Achilles tendon, as such injections can lead to further tendon degeneration and rupture. Patients with persistent symptoms of retrocalcaneal bursitis or Achilles tendinitis, despite 4 to 6 weeks of nonoperative management, should be referred to an orthopaedic consultant for further evaluation and management.

Plantar Fasciitis

Plantar fasciitis is a common condition that is difficult to treat effectively. The physician must counsel the patient that plantar fasciitis often takes many months to completely resolve, that the expected outcome is slow resolution of symptoms during the treatment period. In general, treatment consists of administration of NSAIDs, institution of stretching exercises for the plantar fascia, and use of heel cups in the shoes. In addition the patient should be counseled to wear shoes with a wide heel, a stiff heel counter, a soft, thick sole, and a good arch support. The initial management (NSAIDs, stretching, heel cups) will resolve symptoms within 3 months in nearly 90% of patients with plantar fasciitis. In patients refractory to this treatment, consideration should be given to custom-molded, semirigid, full-length orthotics for the shoes to better support the arch and cushion the heel of the foot. Consideration also should be given to injections of local anesthetics and corticosteroids at the site of maximal tenderness at the origin of the plantar fascia in the heel. The physician should counsel the patient that injections into the heel are extremely painful and are not always successful in relieving symptoms. Consideration should also be given to a trial of casting in patients with severe plantar fasciitis refractory to the usual nonoperative measures. Surgical release rarely is indicated for plantar fasciitis. After 3 months, patients with plantar fasciitis still refractory to treatment should be referred to an orthopaedist for further evaluation and management.

Tarsal Tunnel Syndrome and Posterior Tibial Tendinitis

These conditions are treated with NSAIDs and a short-leg walking cast or a brace that holds the ankle, heel, and foot in neutral alignment throughout gait. Patients refractory to this type of treatment should be referred to an orthopaedic consultant for consideration of more aggressive treatment measures such as corticosteroid injections in the area around the posterior tibial tendon or surgical decompression of the tarsal tunnel.

Tarsal Coalition

Patients with limited subtalar motion or absence of subtalar motion should be referred to an orthopaedic consultant for consideration of nonoperative or operative management.

Sever's Disease

Children with calcaneal apophysitis should be treated symptomatically with NSAIDs, stretching of the Achilles tendon, and heel lifts within the shoes. In severe cases, a trial of short-leg casting is also considered. Children with symptoms refractory to these measures after 4 to 6 weeks of treatment should be referred to an orthopaedic consultant for further evaluation and management.

17

FOOT PAIN

Douglas R. Dirschl

The foot is the platform that supports the body's weight during standing and that moves the body during walking, running, and jumping. Structural abnormalities in the foot, imbalances between the bones and supporting musculature, or abnormal demands placed on the foot may cause foot pain. Pain in the midfoot and forefoot is one of the most common musculoskeletal complaints.

■ PHONE CALL

Questions

1. How long has the pain been present?

The mode of onset and time course of the foot pain can be important clues to the cause of the symptoms. For example, the acute onset of pain, erythema, and swelling at the first metatarsophalangeal (MTP) joint generally is indicative of gout, whereas deformity and the insidious onset of pain at the same joint most commonly is caused by a hallux valgus (bunion) deformity.

2. How old is the patient?

The age of the patient can be helpful in delineating the source of the pain, since the forefoot disorders most common in children are different from the forefoot disorders most common in adults.

3. Is the pain associated with weight bearing alone or is it present at rest as well?

Pain that occurs only with weight bearing generally indicates a structural or functional abnormality in the foot, whereas pain also present at rest may indicate an inflammatory condition, infection, or neurologic disorder.

4. Does the patient have a history of foot disorders?

It is important to know if the patient has a history of foot problems, as prior disorders or prior surgeries may provide important clues to the current diagnosis.

5. Does the patient have a history of other medical problems?

Other medical problems, such as gout or diabetes, frequently are manifest in the foot and may provide important clues to the likely cause of the foot pain.

Orders

None. If infection of the foot is strongly suspected, the physician should consider ordering a CBC and ESR prior to evaluating the patient. Otherwise, laboratory and radiographic studies can be deferred until physical evaluation is completed.

Inform RN

"I will arrive at the bedside/emergency department in 60 minutes." In the absence of injury, pain in the midfoot or forefoot is almost never a medical emergency, and the patient may be evaluated in a reasonable amount of time.

■ ELEVATOR THOUGHTS

- Infectious disorders
    Acute and chronic osteomyelitis
    Septic arthritis
- Inflammatory disorders
    Gout
    Rheumatoid arthritis
- Degenerative conditions
    Osteoarthrosis
    Hallux rigidus
    Freiberg's infraction
- Mechanical disorders
    Hallux valgus
    Pes planus
    Pes cavus
    Hammertoes
    Claw toes
- Neurologic disorders
    Morton's neuroma
    Charcot's arthropathy

■ BEDSIDE

Vital Signs

Vital signs are not necessary in the evaluation of pain in the foot unless infection is strongly suspected.

Selective History

How long have symptoms been present?
    It is important to ascertain the nature of onset and duration of the symptoms. Most mechanical and degenerative conditions of

the foot are characterized by the slow, insidious onset of pain, with progression of symptoms over an extended period. Inflammatory and infectious conditions generally are characterized by a rapid onset of more severe pain.

Does the patient have a history of injuries to or problems of the foot?

It is important to ascertain whether the patient has had foot problems or disorders in the past. A history of gout should lead the physician to suspect a repeat attack of gout, seen most frequently in the first MTP joint. A history of diabetes should lead the physician to suspect ulceration or Charcot's neuropathy. A history of surgery for a painful bunion should lead the physician to suspect pain related to that surgical procedure.

What is the precise location of the pain?

The precise location and nature of the pain should be ascertained also. Pain confined only to the MTP joint of the great toe generally indicates gout, an inflamed bunion, or hallux rigidus. Pain confined to the web space between the third and fourth toes that is associated with numbness or tingling extending to the tips of adjacent toes is characteristic of Morton's neuroma.

What types of shoes does the patient normally wear?

The patient's typical shoe wear should also be ascertained and examined. Claw toes and hammertoes are common but generally are painful only when the patient wears shoes that are too constrictive in the toe box, thus putting excessive pressure on the toes (Fig. 17–1).

Selective Physical Examination

Inspection

The shoes and socks should be removed and both feet and legs exposed to midcalf level. The feet should be inspected and compared for swelling (either generalized or localized), erythema, and shape. The height of the patient's medial longitudinal arch should be examined in each foot without weight bearing and then reexamined with the patient standing. The toes should be examined for evidence of clawing or hammertoe deformity. Similarly, the great toe should be inspected for hallux valgus deformity.

Palpation

All areas around the midfoot and forefoot should be carefully palpated for areas of localized tenderness. Localized tenderness almost always indicates a disorder at that particular site.

Range of Motion

It is difficult to accurately test range of motion of the midfoot, and generally it is not recommended that this be done. Range of

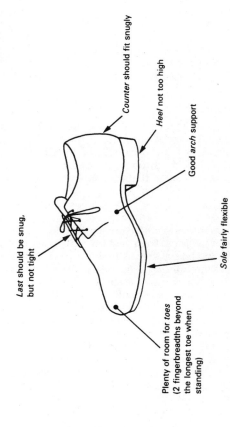

Last should be snug, but not tight

Plenty of room for *toes* (2 fingerbreadths beyond the longest toe when standing)

Sole fairly flexible

Good *arch* support

Heel not too high

Counter should fit snugly

Figure 17–1 □ Features of comfortable, supportive, durable shoes to be recommended to patients. (From Birnbaum JS: The Musculoskeletal Manual, 2nd ed. Philadelphia, WB Saunders, 1986, p 254.)

motion of the MTP and interphalangeal joints should be assessed and recorded. This motion should be compared to that of the asymptomatic foot. In addition, pain on movement of the involved toes should also be sought and recorded.

Special Tests

Hallux rigidus can be diagnosed by restricted range of motion and pain on movement of the great toe MTP joint.

Morton's neuroma (interdigital neuroma) can be diagnosed by pressing or tapping in the intermetatarsal web space between the two involved toes. If this pressure or tapping reproduces the patient's pain, a presumptive diagnosis of Morton's neuroma can be made. In addition, the metatarsal heads can be pressed together in an attempt to reproduce the symptoms. Reproducing the patient's symptoms with this maneuver also leads to a presumptive diagnosis of Morton's neuroma.

Neurologic Examination

Active extension and flexion of the toes should be tested to get a rudimentary determination of strength in the toes. In addition, sensibility in all areas of the foot should be tested and carefully documented. Poor sensibility throughout the foot generally is due to the peripheral neuropathy of diabetes or to a vascular disorder.

Further Orders

Radiographs of the foot should be obtained in nearly all patients complaining of forefoot pain. The standard radiographic series includes AP, oblique, and lateral views of the foot. These radiographs should be examined carefully for deformity, especially in the area of symptoms, as well as for any soft tissue swelling. In addition the MTP and interphalangeal joints should be examined for marginal erosions, which may be indicative of rheumatoid arthritis or gout, and for calcific densities, which may be present in gout and pseudogout. If gout or acute infection of the MTP joint is suspected, the joint should be aspirated with a 22-gauge needle inserted into the MTP joint. Any fluid obtained should be sent for Gram stain and culture, as well as for a cell count and examination for calcium pyrophosphate (pseudogout) or calcium urate (gout) crystals.

If Morton's neuroma is suspected, an injection of local anesthetic into the involved interspace might relieve symptoms and provide further presumptive evidence that the diagnosis of Morton's neuroma is correct.

■ MANAGEMENT

Gout generally is diagnosed either because of a history of gout in the presence of classic signs and symptom or because of the demonstration of urate crystals on joint aspiration. It has been said that gout and septic arthritis never occur simultaneously; therefore the presence of urate crystals on joint aspiration effectively rules out the possibility of septic arthritis. Pseudogout (calcium pyrophosphate crystal disease) and infection can coexist, however, so the physician must still suspect septic arthritis if calcium pyrophosphate crystals are present on aspiration of joint fluid. The goal of treatment of gout is to rapidly reduce the acute inflammation in the first MTP joint. This can be achieved by treatment with elevation and ice, as well as by eliminating alcohol and medications such as aspirin, which elevate serum uric acid levels. Oral colchicine often is used to decrease the pain and inflammation of acute gout. Colchicine 0.6 mg may be given orally each hour until the pain abates or the patient experiences gastrointestinal upset from the medication. Colchicine is then given in twice daily doses of 0.6 mg until symptoms resolve. Allopurinol generally is used in the treatment of chronic gout rather than in the treatment of the acute inflammatory phase of gout. Indomethacin or another NSAID often is effective in the treatment of acute gout. Relieving the pressure on the foot either by supportive shoe wear or crutches also can help decrease symptoms and inflammation. Finally, gout is the archetypal acute inflammatory monarthritis. It may respond dramatically to local injection of a corticosteroid.

Acute osteomyelitis or septic arthritis generally is treated with surgical debridement and administration of antibiotics. Orthopaedic consultation should be obtained in these conditions.

Osteoarthritis of the forefoot generally is treated nonspecifically to help reduce symptoms. Effective measures include NSAIDs and shoes that do not put pressure on the painful area and that have a firm, thick sole to support the foot.

Hallux rigidus is treated initially with NSAIDs and a shoe with a wide and tall toe box and a firm or even rigid sole to relieve pressure on the joint. Continued symptoms or the presence of large osteophytes on radiographs should prompt orthopaedic consultation.

Freiberg's infraction is avascular necrosis and collapse of the second metatarsal head. This condition is treated symptomatically with shoe modifications and anti-inflammatory medications. If symptoms persist beyond 6 to 8 weeks, orthopaedic consultation should be obtained.

Painful flatfoot (pes planus) in the adult seldom requires surgical intervention. Anti-inflammatory medications and a good arch support are generally all that are needed to relieve symptoms. The physician must keep in mind, however, that painful flatfoot often is associated with other foot deformities or conditions. When symptoms do not resolve rapidly with treatment, orthopaedic consultation should be obtained.

Painful pes cavus is uncommon. It usually is treated symptomatically, but orthopaedic consultation in these patients should be obtained, since pes cavus frequently can be a manifestation of other more serious neurologic or mechanical conditions.

The goal in the treatment of hallux valgus (bunion), claw toes, and hammertoes is relief of symptoms. It is important to note that the primary goal in treating these conditions is not restoration of normal appearance to the foot; neither nonoperative nor operative treatment for these conditions should be undertaken with the primary goal of improving the cosmetic appearance of the foot. Basic treatment for these conditions involves NSAIDs to decrease pain and special shoes to relieve areas of increased pressure. Shoes with a firm rubber sole, a wide toe box, and a tall toe box are used most commonly in treating these conditions. In addition, a donut pad over the medial bunion (or the callosity in the case of claw toes) may be helpful. Failure to relieve the pain with these measures should prompt referral to an orthopaedist.

Morton's neuroma usually occurs between the third and fourth toes of the foot. Nonoperative treatment of this condition usually is successful, and surgery rarely is necessary. Nonoperative treatment consists of shoes with a wide toe box to reduce pressure on the metatarsal heads, which may compress the neuroma and worsen symptoms. Injecting the area with a corticosteroid also may relieve symptoms. If the patient fails to respond after 6 to 8 weeks of nonoperative treatment, the patient should be referred to an orthopaedist for consideration of surgical treatment.

18

POSTOPERATIVE PAIN

Douglas R. Dirschl

In the first 24 to 48 hours after orthopaedic surgery, nearly all patients will experience pain in the area operated on. Some degree of postoperative pain and swelling is anticipated and is considered normal. One of the most frequent calls for the orthopaedic house officer, however, is to evaluate the postoperative patient complaining of pain.

■ PHONE CALL

Questions

1. **What surgical procedure did the patient undergo?**

   It is important to know precisely what surgical procedure was performed on the patient; this knowledge will allow the physician to gauge the expected level of postoperative pain as well as to bring to mind any complications commonly associated with that particular surgical procedure.

2. **When was the surgical procedure performed?**

   Most patients have the greatest pain in the first 24 hours following the operation. Therefore, knowing how long it has been since the surgery is important in gauging how much postoperative pain can be expected.

3. **What medications is the patient receiving?**

   One common source of excessive postoperative pain is inadequate postoperative analgesia. The patient's current regimen of postoperative analgesics should be ascertained to determine whether it is adequate for the expected level of postoperative pain.

4. **What is the neurovascular status of the operated-on extremity?**

   It is important to assess the neurologic and vascular status of the operated-on limb in all patients complaining of postoperative pain. Swelling and compartment syndrome following surgery are possible sources of the pain and should be ruled out in every patient.

Orders

None.

Inform RN

"I will arrive at the bedside in 15 to 30 minutes." Postoperative pain in a patient generally does not warrant emergency evaluation, but all patients with excessive postoperative pain should be evaluated urgently to rule out potentially serious surgical complications.

■ ELEVATOR THOUGHTS

- Inadequate postoperative analgesia
- Postoperative edema
- Postoperative infection
- Compartment syndrome
- Failure of surgical stabilization
- Exaggerated pain response
- Chronic pain behavior

■ BEDSIDE

Vital Signs

Vital signs should be ascertained frequently in all patients in the postoperative period. If a patient complaining of severe postoperative pain does not have the normal physiologic responses to pain (tachycardia and hypertension), the physician should suspect chronic pain behavior.

Selective History

What surgical procedure was performed and when was it performed?

It is important to know precisely what surgical procedure was performed and when it was performed. The hospital chart should be scrutinized to determine the precise surgical procedure, as well as any intraoperative irregularities or complications. If implants were inserted, the evaluating physician should know what implants were inserted and at what location. Although uncommon in the early postoperative period, implant failure can be a source of postoperative pain.

What is the precise location of the patient's pain?

It is necessary to know the precise location of the patient's pain to determine its relationship to the surgical procedure performed and to make decisions regarding pain management.

Selective Physical Examination

Inspection

The operated-on limb should be inspected for swelling and erythema. Soft dressings should be fully removed to expose the injured limb. If a cast or splint has been applied, it should not be removed at the initial evaluation but removed later if deemed truly necessary. The surgical incisions should be inspected for swelling, erythema, and drainage.

Palpation

The area surrounding the surgical incision should be gently palpated for tenderness and swelling. The physician must remember that tenderness surrounding a surgical incision nearly always is present in the first 48 hours after surgery. Excessive tenderness, however, or a collection of fluid beneath the skin may indicate infection or a hematoma. Massive swelling and tightness of the limb may indicate impending compartment syndrome.

Range of Motion

The toes or fingers should be moved through active and passive ranges of motion. Some pain with passive range of motion of the digits is to be expected because of postoperative swelling more proximal in the extremity. Severe pain in the forearm or leg on passive movement of the fingers or toes, however, may indicate impending compartment syndrome.

Neurologic and Vascular Examination

Capillary refill time and warmth of the fingers or toes should be assessed. Cool digits or capillary refill time in excess of 2 seconds may indicate sluggish vascular inflow to the extremity. In the most severe case, however, it may indicate compartment syndrome.

Sensibility should be carefully tested over the entire operated-on limb. Globally decreased sensibility may be related to swelling and increased pressure within the limb. More commonly, however, this finding is related to intraoperative use of a tourniquet, which has led to a temporary hypoesthesia in the entire limb distal to the tourniquet. In the absence of any signs of impending compartment syndrome, globally decreased sensibility probably is due to a tourniquet palsy. Decreased sensibility in the distribution of a specific peripheral nerve likely is due to minor injury to that nerve during the operative procedure.

Further Orders

If infection or hematoma is suspected, a CBC and ESR are in order. If hardware failure or dislocation of an operated-on joint is suspected, radiographs should be obtained immediately. Although not entirely reliable, pulse oximetry applied to the digits in the involved extremity may be helpful; oxygen saturation in the involved extremity greater than 90% generally indicates adequate vascular inflow.

■ MANAGEMENT

In the absence of signs of infection, hematoma, or impending compartment syndrome, no specific management of the operated-on limb is necessary. The patient's postoperative analgesic medications should be carefully reviewed, however, to ensure that they are adequate to control the expected amount of postoperative pain. For example, oral analgesics in the first 24 hours following major surgery generally are not effective; the patient often is nauseated and somewhat obtunded during recovery from general anesthesia and is not able to take oral pain medications. Parenteral analgesics usually are much more effective in the immediate postoperative period in these patients. The physician should not always assume that because an analgesic order was written the patient received the medication. The medication flow sheet should be reviewed to ensure the patient is receiving adequate doses of analgesic medications.

Sedatives and hypnotics generally are not indicated in the management of immediate postoperative pain. These medications can be dangerous, especially when administered in concert with narcotic analgesics, and should be avoided in the early postoperative period. Similarly, elderly patients are sensitive to all medications, and analgesic and hypnotic medications in the elderly should be kept to the minimum necessary to control postoperative pain.

If infection or hematoma is suspected, an orthopaedic surgeon should be consulted regarding further management. This may consist of antibiotics, observation, aspiration, or return to the operating room for reexploration.

Swelling in the limb probably is one of the most common causes of postoperative pain. Generally this is managed by elevation of the limb, removal of all constricting dressings, and administration of appropriate analgesic medication. If postoperative swelling is suspected as the cause of pain, orthopaedic consultation should be obtained to loosen the splint or bivalve the cast on the involved extremity.

The management of acute compartment syndrome is discussed in Chapter 32.

If, after thorough evaluation, no cause can be determined for the patient's complaints of excessive postoperative pain, it is possible that the patient is exhibiting chronic pain behavior. This is especially true with patients who have a history of substance abuse, particularly narcotic abuse. In this situation the patient should be reassured that the postoperative pain is at the expected level, that the limb is not at risk, and that there will be no devastating complications during the postoperative period. A combination of firm reassurance, appropriate analgesic medications, and elevation are generally successful in managing these patients.

19

POSTOPERATIVE NUMBNESS

Douglas R. Dirschl

Although not common, postoperative numbness in the extremities can occur for a variety of reasons. In most cases the loss of sensibility is incomplete and transient and will resolve with observation alone. However, the physician must be able to recognize sources of numbness that will not resolve spontaneously, initiate the appropriate management, and counsel the patient as to the expected outcome.

■ PHONE CALL

Questions

1. **What surgical procedure did the patient undergo and when was the surgical procedure performed?**
   Knowledge of the precise surgical procedure performed as well as of the time interval since the operation can aid the physician in determining the source of the patient's numbness. For example, surgical stabilization of a humeral shaft fracture can result in injury to the radial nerve in the arm, which would cause weakness in wrist and finger extension and numbness over the dorsoradial border of the hand.
2. **What is the precise location of the patient's numbness?**
   It is necessary to know the particular site of the numbness to determine its cause. Numbness throughout the extremity likely is due to tourniquet palsy, whereas numbness in a specific peripheral nerve distribution most likely is due to a contusion or injury to that particular nerve.
3. **What is the vascular status of the patient's limb?**
   Determining the vascular status of the operated-on extremity is important. Impaired vascularity, due to vascular disruption or to severe swelling, will result in paresthesias throughout the area of poor vascular inflow.

Orders

None.

Inform RN

"I will arrive at the bedside in less than 15 minutes." Although most numbness in the postoperative period is transient and there is full recovery, these patients should be evaluated immediately to exclude other irreversible causes of postoperative numbness.

■ ELEVATOR THOUGHTS

- Tourniquet palsy
- Peripheral nerve contusion
- Compartment syndrome
- Postoperative use of local or regional anesthetics

■ BEDSIDE

Vital Signs

Vital signs usually are not necessary in the evaluation of patients with postoperative numbness. Good vascularity of the limb must be documented, however, to rule out dysvascularity as a cause of the numbness.

Selective History

What surgical procedure was performed and when was it performed?

The physician should begin his or her evaluation by looking at the patient's chart to gain as much information as possible about the surgical procedure. It is important to know precisely what surgical procedure was performed and what surgical approach was used. Knowledge of the common orthopaedic approaches and their relationship to nearby nerves aids in diagnosing the cause of the numbness.

Was a tourniquet used during the surgical procedure?

It is important to know whether an extremity tourniquet was used during the surgical procedure and, if so, how long and to what pressure it was inflated. Inflation of the tourniquet to pressures over 300 mm Hg for longer than 2 hours is associated with transient postoperative tourniquet palsy.

Was a postoperative local or regional anesthesia administered in the operating room?

Surgeons commonly infiltrate surgical sites with a long-acting local anesthetic to provide postoperative analgesia. In these cases, postoperative numbness simply may be due to the effects of this local anesthetic. Similarly, epidural or interscalene blocks may be administered by an anesthesiologist for postoperative analgesia of the lower and upper limb, respectively. The physician must be familiar with these local and regional blocks to fully assess the patient with postoperative numbness.

At the bedside the physician should inquire of the patient the specific location of the numbness, searching for clues as to whether it involves a single peripheral nerve or a larger portion of the operated-on extremity. The patient should be asked if there is pain associated with the numbness. Pain associated with postoperative numbness and massive swelling of the operated-on limb may indicate impending compartment syndrome.

Selective Physical Examination

Inspection and Palpation

The physician should perform a careful vascular examination to determine whether the vascular inflow to the operated-on extremity is adequate. Palpating pulses and assessing capillary refill time in the fingers or toes are often all that are necessary in this regard. In a normally perfused limb the capillary refill time will be less than 2 seconds. The limb should also be palpated for swelling and tenseness, and the fingers or toes should be put through a passive range of motion. A swollen, tense limb with poor capillary refill time and severe pain on passive motion of the fingers or toes may indicate compartment syndrome (see Chapter 32).

Neurologic Examination

A careful neurologic examination should be performed, focusing on both motor and sensory components of the examination. It is important to differentiate between a purely sensory neurologic deficit and one that involves the motor nerves as well. For discussions of the dermatomal distribution of peripheral sensibility and careful manual motor testing for the upper and lower extremities the reader is directed to texts dealing with physical evaluation and anatomy.

Further Orders

Generally no further orders are necessary.

■ MANAGEMENT

Tourniquet Palsy

Tourniquet palsy is characterized by global hypoesthesias in the extremity distal to the site of the intraoperative tourniquet. The symptoms of tourniquet palsy may be burning paresthesias or numbness. These symptoms occur more frequently when the tourniquet is inflated for a prolonged period during the operative procedure. The management of tourniquet palsy consists of reassuring the patient that symptoms are transient and observing carefully for return of sensory function. Motor function is affected infrequently by tourniquet palsy.

Peripheral Nerve Injury

Peripheral nerve injury from a surgical procedure is almost always a neurapraxia: the nerve is stretched or contused either during surgical retraction or because of the inflammation following the surgical procedure. Neurapraxias usually are transient and generally do not necessitate immediate surgical reexploration. Nerve lacerations can also occur, however, and it is advisable to consult the orthopaedic surgeon or another member of the surgical team in cases of peripheral nerve dysfunction following an operation. The patient's surgeon will know best whether the surgical approach was dangerously near the involved peripheral nerve.

Compartment Syndrome

The evaluation and management of acute compartment syndrome are discussed in detail in Chapter 32.

Administration of Postoperative Local or Regional Anesthetics

Postoperative numbness due to the administration of local or regional anesthetic at the conclusion of the surgical procedure is always transient, resolving completely when the anesthetic effect has worn off. The patient should simply be reassured that the postoperative numbness is due to the administration of postoperative anesthetic and that sensibility will return spontaneously when the medication has worn off.

PROBLEMS WITH ASSOCIATED TRAUMA

20

BASIC PRINCIPLES OF MUSCULOSKELETAL TRAUMA

C. Michael LeCroy

Injuries to the musculoskeletal system represent the orthopaedic conditions most commonly encountered clinically. Injuries to the neck, back, and extremities account for millions of emergency department and outpatient clinic visits each year, as well as for countless hospital admissions and work-loss days. Musculoskeletal injuries range in severity from simple sprains and contusions to fractures of multiple extremities. Each type of orthopaedic injury (or constellation of injuries) is associated with a characteristic morbidity and disability. Early intervention and consultation is indicated in all cases to assure optimal opportunity for healing and restoration of function.

Initial evaluation and preliminary treatment of most orthopaedic traumatic conditions are rendered by a nonorthopaedist. This initial assessment and management take place most commonly in the emergency department or outpatient clinic setting. An important component of this initial evaluation is the *history;* i.e., how did the injury occur? An understanding of the mechanism of trauma can alert the physician to certain types of orthopaedic injuries. For example, a patient who is seen after having his leg crushed by a moving car is at significant risk for developing a compartment syndrome. Similarly, patients seen after high-speed motor vehicle crashes will be expected to have more significant soft tissue and bone trauma than patients seen after simple falls or sports-related injuries.

Once an accurate history has been obtained, a thorough *physical examination* should be the next step. Depending on information obtained from the history, this examination often can be focused on the obvious problem at hand, e.g., the patient's swollen ankle. In situations in which the patient has sustained injuries from a high-energy force, however, it is imperative to systematically examine the entire musculoskeletal system. This is necessary to minimize the chance of missing injuries that might not be immediately obvious. It is easy for the physician and other health care providers to become distracted by the obvious open fracture of the femur and in so doing miss the more subtle tarsometatarsal dislocations of the contralateral foot.

Examination of the injured extremity (or spine) should always follow a basic sequence. First, the extremity is *visually inspected* for deformity, skin and soft tissue integrity, swelling, and ecchymosis or other discoloration. Then the extremity is *palpated,* and areas of tenderness in the soft tissues, joints, and bony prominences are identified. The *vascular status* of the extremity is assessed next by palpation or Doppler evaluation of distal pulses. Finally, *neurologic function* is tested via a focused motor, sensory, and reflex examination. The importance of a careful and accurate neurovascular assessment during this initial examination cannot be overemphasized. In far too many cases, "WNL" (within normal limits) listed on this part of the examination form has meant "We Never Looked."

Once the injured extremity, neck, or spine has been examined, the next step in the assessment of the injured orthopaedic patient is to obtain pertinent *radiographs.* The type and number of radiographs ordered are determined by the results of the history and physical examination. As a general rule, two radiographic views in separate (orthogonal) planes should be obtained for evaluation of extremity trauma. This most commonly translates into AP and lateral images. Often, consultation with an orthopaedist is advisable to ensure that adequate radiographs are obtained to confirm or rule out suspected trauma. The radiographs are reviewed, and the presence or absence of fracture or joint dislocation is identified.

If a musculoskeletal injury (sprain, joint dislocation, or fracture) is identified as a result of the above assessment, the physician should next take steps to *protect the injured extremity(ies).* These techniques were described in detail in Chapter 4. The principles of extremity protection can be remembered easily by the pneumonic PRICE:

P: Protection of extremity, usually via splinting

R: Rest for extremity to avoid further injury and pain

I: Ice or cold therapy to control swelling

C: Compression to injured area, usually in association with splinting

E: Elevation of injured extremity above heart level

It is important to remember that to prevent further damage, the extremity (or spine) can and should be protected at any point in the evaluation of the injured patient that an injury becomes apparent. For example, the patient with an obviously deformed thigh should not be sent to radiology with his or her femur fracture unsplinted.

Most injuries to the musculoskeletal system are evaluated initially by a nonorthopaedist. Many simple injuries (e.g., sprains and strains) can and should be managed without immediate *orthopaedic consultation;* however, many injuries do require urgent orthopaedic evaluation and treatment to optimize outcome. Unfortunately there are no hard-and-fast rules regarding when it is necessary to consult the orthopaedic specialist. With the exception of orthopaedic emergent conditions (as outlined in Chapter 5), in which consultation is indicated in all cases, the decision to obtain immediate orthopaedic consultation must be made on a case-by-case basis. Multiple factors enter into this decision, including the severity of the injury, the experience of the treating physician, and the availability of the orthopaedic specialist. As a general rule, the orthopaedist should be consulted for all fractures and major joint dislocations. Often the orthopaedic consultant can provide input to direct the radiographic examination of the patient as well as the initial immobilization of the injured extremity. When in doubt, it is prudent for the treating physician to request orthopaedic consultation. This policy will ensure that all significant orthopaedic traumatic conditions get appropriate initial treatment.

To summarize, a systematic evaluation of the patient with suspected musculoskeletal trauma is necessary. The principles discussed are applicable to simple orthopaedic injuries as well as to complex multiple-extremity trauma. Injuries to the musculoskeletal system should be evaluated using this sequence of steps:

1. History of injury
2. Physical examination
3. Radiographic examination
4. Protection of extremity
5. Orthopaedic consultation, where indicated

Following these steps will enable the initial treating physician to correctly identify and initially manage most significant injuries to the musculoskeletal system.

■ TYPES OF MUSCULOSKELETAL TRAUMATIC CONDITIONS

The musculoskeletal system can experience a wide variety of injuries, ranging in severity from simple contusions to complex periarticular fractures. A familiarity with the various types of injuries is necessary for adequate assessment of the injured back and extremities. In addition, an understanding of these different injuries will allow the treating physician to appropriately triage musculoskeletal injuries, including consultation with the orthopaedic specialist.

It is important for the clinician to remember that musculoskeletal trauma includes injury to the soft tissues of the axial skeleton and extremities as well as injury to bones and joints. Injured patients frequently will present with **contusion,** which is an indication of trauma to the skin and underlying soft tissue structures. Contusions, which usually are associated with tenderness and swelling, can be an indicator of more significant injury to the extremity than might first be appreciated. In general a painful contusion following trauma warrants radiographic evaluation of the extremity to rule out associated bone injury.

Laceration is another important finding on the musculoskeletal examination. This disruption in the integrity of the skin is a direct indication of soft tissue trauma. It is critical to remember that a complete neurovascular examination is particularly important with an extremity laceration. Depending on the location and depth of the laceration, underlying neurologic, vascular, and musculotendinous structures may be involved. To preserve limb function, these injuries must be identified and treated expeditiously. A laceration also increases the risk of infection. This is particularly true for lacerations that communicate directly with joints (intraarticular communication) or with fractures (open fractures). The management of extremity lacerations varies with the location, depth, level of contamination, age of injury, and the possibility of associated fracture or joint involvement. Complex lacerations, including those associated with fracture and intraarticular extension, should be managed in conjunction with the orthopaedic specialist.

A third group of soft tissue injuries to the musculoskeletal system includes sprains and strains, two terms frequently confused with one another. A **sprain** refers specifically to injury to a joint ligament. The most common orthopaedic injury seen in emergency departments and outpatient clinics is the ankle sprain. The hallmark of sprains is swelling and tenderness in the area of the joint following injury. The diagnosis of sprain generally cannot be made until fracture has been ruled out with appropriate radiographs. Sprains range in severity and prognosis. Most sprains, however, can be treated successfully using the principles of PRICE.

Strain implies trauma to the muscle-tendon units of the spine or extremities. In contrast to sprains, strain injuries do not involve trauma to joints. Muscle strains are also among the most commonly encountered musculoskeletal injuries. For example, in most patients with a diagnosis of cervical whiplash following a motor vehicle accident the cervical paraspinal musculature has been strained. The diagnosis of strain cannot be made until bone and ligament injury have been excluded. The treatment of strains generally is symptomatic; however, recovery can be prolonged, much to the dismay of the patient and the physician alike.

Another type of commonly encountered orthopaedic trauma is **dislocation.** This injury refers specifically to complete displacement of two articular surfaces relative to each other. Frequently dislocation is immediately obvious, as with elbow or shoulder dislocations. In other cases the diagnosis is more subtle, as with carpal or midfoot dislocations. Dislocations can be, and frequently are, associated with periarticular fractures (fracture-dislocation). This determination usually can be made at the time of radiographic confirmation of the diagnosis of joint dislocation. A joint dislocation constitutes an orthopaedic emergency (see Chapter 5). Immediate consultation with an orthopaedic specialist generally is indicated. Delay in treatment (i.e., joint reduction) can increase morbidity and loss of function significantly.

The final type of injury to the musculoskeletal system is **fracture.** In simplest terms, fracture implies disruption in the integrity of the bone. The diagnosis of fracture is suspected from clinical findings and confirmed by appropriate radiographic evaluation of the injured bone or joint. Fractures are described further by terminology such as *displacement, angulation, comminution,* or *intraarticular extension.* See Chapter 2 for definitions of the terms commonly used to characterize fracture patterns.

Chapters 21 to 35 address the orthopaedic conditions commonly associated with trauma. As in Section I, the conditions will be discussed on a regional anatomic basis. These chapters highlight the most frequently encountered injuries (i.e., strains, sprains, dislocations, and fractures) and delineate the appropriate initial evaluation and management of these conditions.

21

NECK PAIN

C. Michael LeCroy

The region of the neck can be injured in a variety of ways. Motor vehicle accidents continue to be the primary source of most such injuries. Neck injuries, however, also can be caused by falls or recreational accidents. Neck injuries range in severity from muscle strains (cervical whiplash) to complex fracture-dislocations of the cervical spine. Fortunately most cervical injuries are not associated with any neurologic deficit. Because of the potential for devastating neurologic sequelae, however, any patient with suspected cervical trauma must have his or her cervical spine adequately immobilized until fracture, dislocation, or ligament injury has been ruled out radiographically. All complaints of neck pain following high-energy trauma must be taken seriously, and urgent evaluation is indicated in all cases.

■ PHONE CALL

Questions

1. **How was the neck injured?**
    An understanding of the mechanism of injury is critical in the evaluation of musculoskeletal trauma. This is the initial step in the formulation of a differential diagnosis.
2. **Can the patient localize the pain?**
    The ability of the patient to localize the pain to a specific region can be helpful in establishing a diagnosis. Not uncommonly, however, patients with neck trauma will present with diffuse pain.
3. **Can the patient move all four extremities?**
    Spontaneous or voluntary movements of the extremities can provide a rough assessment of whether there is concomitant neurologic injury. A complete neurologic evaluation must be performed subsequently during physical examination of the patient.
4. **Does the patient complain of numbness or tingling in the hands or feet?**
    Radicular-like symptoms of radiating pain and intermittent tingling can be signs of nerve root involvement.
5. **Has the cervical spine been immobilized?**
    The cervical spine should be protected pending clinical and

radiographic evaluation in patients complaining of posttraumatic neck pain, particularly following high-energy trauma.

6. **Does the patient have any associated injuries?**

As with all trauma to the musculoskeletal system, associated injuries to the axial skeleton as well as to other body systems must be excluded. This is particularly important for high-energy trauma, in which the incidence of associated injuries is high.

7. **Is the patient hemodynamically stable?**

Hemodynamic stability is the first priority of management in all trauma victims. If the patient is not hemodynamically stable, attention should be turned to the ABCs (airway, breathing, and circulation) before the musculoskeletal injury is evaluated.

Orders

1. If the neck has not been immobilized previously, take immediate steps to ensure that the cervical spine is protected adequately in all patients who have sustained trauma to the neck. Most commonly this involves application of a rigid cervical collar. In the absence of this type of cervical orthosis, rolled sheets or sandbags may be placed to each side of the neck to immobilize the cervical spine.

2. If the patient has sustained a high-energy mechanism of injury, such as a motor vehicle accident, ask the RN to obtain immediate consultation with a trauma specialist (emergency medicine physician or general surgeon).

Inform RN

"I will arrive at the bedside/emergency department immediately."

Neck injuries require that the patient be seen and evaluated immediately because of the potential for neurologic sequelae and the high incidence of associated injuries.

■ ELEVATOR THOUGHTS

Strains
- Cervical whiplash (paraspinal muscle injury)
- Trapezius strain

Sprains
- Cervical spine ligament injury

Dislocations
- Facet dislocation
    unilateral
    bilateral

Fractures

- Upper cervical spine
  Jefferson fracture (ring of C1)
  Odontoid (dens) fracture (odontoid process of C2)
  Hangman's fracture (pedicles of C2)
- Lower cervical spine
  Teardrop fracture (anteroinferior margin of vertebral body)
  Vertebral body fracture
  Spinous process fracture

■ BEDSIDE

Quick Look Test

Does the patient look well (comfortable), sick (uncomfortable or distressed), or critical (about to die)?

Patients who have sustained trauma to the neck may have other associated and potentially life-threatening injuries. Patients with neck pain following trauma are almost always distressed and in varying degrees of pain. A quick observation of the supine patient can be helpful in detecting spontaneous movements of the extremities.

Vital Signs

Complete vital signs are essential in evaluating the patient with injury to the neck to ascertain hemodynamic status. In addition, monitoring of vital signs should be ongoing during the initial evaluation in any patient who has been the victim of high-energy trauma. As in the evaluation of all injuries, the **ABC**s are critical:

A: maintain *a*irway

B: ensure adequate *b*reathing/respirations

C: ensure adequate *c*irculation

Selective History

How exactly was the neck injured?

Once hemodynamic stability has been assured, a more detailed assessment of the mechanism of injury can be undertaken. In the case of neck pain following a motor vehicle accident, the physician should attempt to determine the particulars of the injury: How did the accident occur? Was the patient driver or passenger? Front seat or back seat? Was the patient restrained? Was the patient ejected from the vehicle? These details can alert the physician to certain injury patterns. For example, patients in vehicles struck from behind are at increased risk for cervical whiplash injury. Similarly, unrestrained victims of vehicular trauma are at increased risk for blunt injury to the head and neck area with potential for cervical fracture or dislocation.

What was the condition of the patient immediately following the injury?

It is also helpful to determine the status of the patient immediately following the accident or injury: Was the patient conscious throughout? Was the patient moving spontaneously at the scene? Was the patient ambulatory? This information can help establish the potential for significant injury to the cervical spine. A history of loss of consciousness should alert the physician to the potential for serious injury to the head and neck, as well as to other body systems. In contrast, a history of ambulation following the injury makes the possibility of significant neurologic injury unlikely. If the patient is unable to provide this information, it often can be obtained from witnesses to the accident or from emergency medical personnel.

What are the patient-specific factors?

In addition to the particular details of the current injury, it is important to determine whether the patient has any history of cervical spine trauma or degenerative disease. This will allow acute trauma to be distinguished from preexisting problems. The presence of any comorbid factors or chronic medical conditions also should be determined during this portion of the evaluation.

Selective Physical Examination

Inspection

Often much information can be gained by simply observing the patient lying supine. This allows the examiner to assess the degree of discomfort that the patient is experiencing. A rigid neck is an indicator of acute trauma with at least muscle injury. The patient also should be observed for movement. Patients without neurologic injury almost always will be noted to move all four extremities spontaneously, regardless of associated injuries.

Palpation

Many victims of trauma arrive in the emergency department with their cervical spine immobilized in the field because of the potential for cervical spine injury. A significant number of these patients will report no neck pain during their initial evaluation. In these patients it is acceptable to briefly remove the front of the cervical collar and gently palpate the posterior neck region for tenderness. The spinous processes of the cervical spine should be palpated initially, followed by the paraspinal musculature. Even in the absence of tenderness the collar should not be definitively removed until the cervical spine has been cleared radiographically. In patients who complain of neck pain, it is best to leave the collar intact pending review of the initial radiographs.

Because of the high incidence of associated injuries (musculoskeletal and other body systems) with cervical trauma, it is imperative that all patients with suspected neck trauma undergo a systematic examination with palpation from head to toe during the initial evaluation to rule out such injuries.

Neurologic Examination

All victims of neck trauma must have a complete neurologic examination. This should include evaluation of motor, sensory, and reflex function. It is relatively easy for the examiner to rule out major neurologic injury such as quadriplegia or paraplegia, but it is often difficult to accurately diagnose more subtle neurologic injury. A systematic examination of both upper extremities is necessary to assess integrity of cervical nerve root function. Motor function should be graded using the standard scheme (Table 21–1). The following list describes the major motor, sensory, and reflex functions of the nerve roots in the upper extremities:

C5 *motor:* elbow flexion
   sensory: lateral aspect of arm
   reflex: biceps
C6 *motor:* wrist extension
   sensory: radial aspect of forearm and thumb and index fingers
   reflex: brachioradialis
C7 *motor:* wrist flexion, elbow extension
   sensory: long finger
   reflex: triceps
C8 *motor:* finger flexion
   sensory: ulnar aspect of forearm and ring and small fingers
   reflex: none
T1 *motor:* finger abduction and adduction
   sensory: medial aspect of elbow
   reflex: none

Table 21–1 □ MOTOR FUNCTION GRADING

Grade	Description
5	Normal
4	Muscle contraction with full range of motion against gravity with some resistance
3	Muscle contraction with full range of motion against gravity
2	Muscle contraction with full range of motion with gravity eliminated
1	Flicker of muscle contraction
0	No activity

■ FURTHER ORDERS

All patients who have sustained an injury to the neck region must undergo radiographic evaluation of the cervical spine. A standard cervical spine trauma series includes AP, lateral, open mouth, and oblique views. The open mouth, or odontoid, view is helpful in the diagnosis of fractures of the odontoid process of C2 as well as of fractures of the lateral masses of C1. The oblique views are helpful in the evaluation of facet injuries and dislocations. All these views can and should be obtained with the cervical collar in place.

An adequate radiographic examination of the cervical spine requires visualization of the C7–T1 disk space. If this level cannot be seen on the lateral view, an additional view, such as a swimmer's, is indicated. If the C7–T1 disk space cannot be seen on plain radiographs, a CT scan of the cervical spine may be indicated. In general the decision to order this study should be made by the treating trauma physician or spine specialist.

It is important to understand that plain radiographs of the cervical spine are helpful only in the diagnosis of fracture and dislocation; they cannot rule out ligament injury. Many patients will have posterior neck pain despite negative plain films. In these patients, flexion-extension lateral films are indicated to rule out ligament disruption. Flexion-extension radiographs should not be obtained before consultation with a trauma or spine specialist.

■ MANAGEMENT

All complaints of neck pain following trauma must be taken seriously. The cervical spine must be protected adequately during the examination and radiographic evaluation. The purpose of these precautions and procedures is to protect against the possibility of neurologic injury with an unstable cervical injury. As a general rule the safest course of action is to have the cervical spine "cleared" by a trauma specialist or spine specialist (orthopaedist or neurosurgeon). This must be an individual experienced in the interpretation of cervical spine films and the treatment of potential injuries to the bone and ligament structures of the neck. Orthopaedic or neurosurgical consultation should be sought immediately for all patients with abnormalities on radiographs or with abnormal neurologic examination results. Occasionally the consultant will recommend additional radiographic evaluation of the cervical spine to better delineate the injury pattern. This may include a CT scan, an MRI scan, or myelography. In short, early consultation is indicated in the evaluation of neck pain following trauma to assure appropriate identification and treatment of cervical spine injuries.

Facet dislocations of the cervical spine occur following flexion injuries with distraction and rotation. Unilateral facet dislocations generally involve 25% displacement of adjacent vertebrae, whereas bilateral facet dislocations characteristically involve 50% displacement (Fig. 21–1). These injuries are unstable and may be associated with neurologic deficit. Management consists of reduction (traction vs. open reduction) and immobilization (halo ring and vest vs. surgical fusion).

Fracture of the C1 ring (Jefferson fracture) results from an axial load injury. These injuries rarely are associated with neurologic

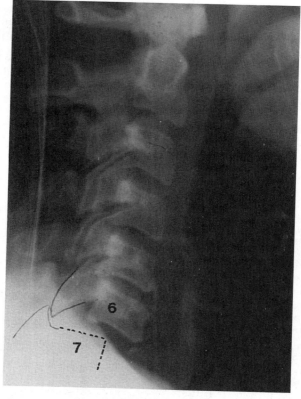

Figure 21–1 □ Lateral cervical spine radiograph, illustrating bilateral facet dislocation at the C6–7 level. Note the anterior displacement of the C6 vertebra by >50%. (From Browner BD, Jupiter JB, Levine AM, Trafton PG [Eds]: Skeletal Trauma. Philadelphia, WB Saunders, 1992, vol 1, p 703.)

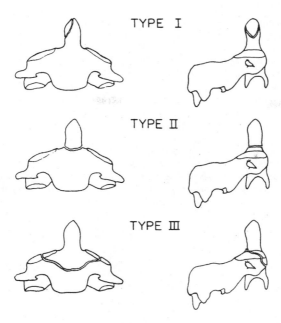

TYPE I

TYPE II

TYPE III

Figure 21–2 □ The classification of odontoid fractures. Type II fractures at the base of the odontoid are associated with a high incidence of displacement and nonunion. (From Anderson LD, D'Alonzo RT: Fractures of the odontoid process of the axis. J Bone Joint Surg (Am) 56:1664, 1974.)

deficit; however, they should be considered unstable and are managed in most cases with halo traction and immobilization. Fractures of C2 may involve the odontoid process (dens fracture) or the isthmus (hangman's fracture). Dens fractures are classified on the basis of the location of the fracture through the odontoid process. Of these injuries, type II fractures at the base of the odontoid process may be particularly problematic because of the potential for displacement and nonunion (Fig. 21–2). The classification and treatment of hangman's fractures are dictated by the amount of displacement. While nondisplaced fractures may be managed in a cervical orthosis, displaced fractures require halo reduction and immobilization.

Fractures of the lower cervical spine involving the vertebral body (teardrop fractures, burst fractures) commonly are unstable and involve neurologic injury. These fractures usually are managed with operative stabilization. In contrast, fractures of the spinous processes of the lower cervical vertebrae, commonly known as clay shoveler's fractures, are stable injuries and require only symptomatic treatment.

Fortunately most cases of neck pain following trauma do not involve significant bone or ligament injury. In these cases, paraspinal muscle or trapezius strain usually is implicated. Once the cervical spine has been cleared radiographically, attention can be directed to symptomatic treatment of the muscle strain. As described for nontraumatic neck pain, narcotic analgesics generally should be avoided, as their use often results in dependency. Pharmacologic treatment instead should consist of NSAIDs as well as mild antispasmodic agents for patients with significant muscle spasm. Application of heat to the posterior neck muscles often is helpful, and a structured physical therapy program for stretching and muscle strengthening should be initiated as soon as possible. A soft cervical collar may be used temporarily for relief of symptoms; however, prolonged collar wear is not advisable, as this may actually weaken the paraspinal musculature.

22

SHOULDER PAIN

C. Michael LeCroy

The shoulder is one of the most complex and frequently injured joints in the body. Shoulder function depends on the coordinated movements of the glenohumeral, acromioclavicular, sternoclavicular, and scapulothoracic articulations (Fig. 22–1). An extensive and complex range of motion is possible in the shoulder, and for this reason the shoulder is particularly susceptible to complications of injury such as stiffness and pain. Furthermore, as testimony to its inherent instability, the glenohumeral joint is the most commonly dislocated joint in the body. Pain in the shoulder region following trauma may reflect injury to one of a number of anatomic structures. Injury to the shoulder occurs frequently in recreational accidents as well as in high-energy mechanisms such as motor vehicle accidents.

■ PHONE CALL

Questions

1. **How was the shoulder injured?**

    An understanding of the mechanism of injury is critical in the evaluation of musculoskeletal trauma. This is the first step in the formulation of a differential diagnosis.

2. **Is there gross deformity?**

    Obvious deformity of the shoulder region usually indicates fracture or dislocation.

3. **Can the patient localize the pain?**

    The ability of the patient to localize the pain to a specific region can be helpful in establishing a diagnosis. Not uncommonly, however, patients with shoulder trauma will present with diffuse pain.

4. **Is there an associated skin wound or laceration?**

    An open wound should alert the physician to the potential for an open fracture or intraarticular communication. These conditions require urgent evaluation and treatment.

5. **Is the patient moving the extremity spontaneously?**

    Spontaneous or voluntary movements of the extremity distal to the site of injury can provide a rough assessment of the presence or absence of concomitant neurologic injury. This must be evaluated subsequently by physical examination.

6. **Does the patient complain of numbness or tingling in the affected upper extremity?**

133

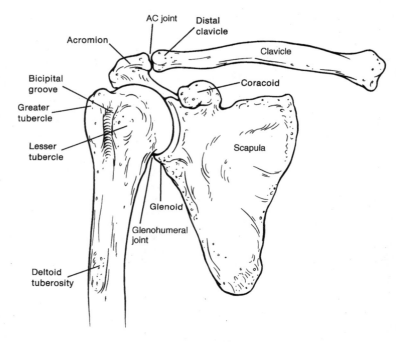

Figure 22–1 □ The skeletal anatomy of the shoulder. (From Wiesel SW, Delahay JN: Essentials of Orthopaedic Surgery, 2nd ed. Philadelphia, WB Saunders, 1997, p 228.)

Radicular-like symptoms of radiating pain and intermittent tingling can signal brachial plexus involvement.

7. Are there any additional injuries?

Associated injuries to the musculoskeletal system as well as to other body systems must be excluded. This is particularly important for high-energy trauma, in which the incidence of associated injuries is high.

8. Is the patient hemodynamically stable?

Hemodynamic stability is the first priority of management in all trauma victims. If the patient is not hemodynamically stable, attention should be turned to the ABCs (airway, breathing, and circulation) before the musculoskeletal injury is evaluated.

Orders

1. To provide the patient as much pain relief as possible and to prevent further damage, ask the RN to immobilize the shoul-

der with a shoulder sling or by strapping the affected arm to the patient's side.

2. If the patient has sustained a high-energy mechanism of injury, such as a motor vehicle accident, ask the RN to obtain immediate consultation with a general trauma specialist (emergency medicine physician or general surgeon).

Inform RN

"I will arrive at the bedside/emergency department within 30 minutes."

In the absence of associated organ system injuries, injury to the shoulder is not usually life or limb threatening. If an open fracture or dislocation is suspected from the described injury mechanism and history, however, the patient should be evaluated on an urgent basis. In general, to minimize patient discomfort and optimize outcome, all injuries to the shoulder should be evaluated as soon as possible.

■ ELEVATOR THOUGHTS

- Strains
    Trapezius strain
- Sprains
    None
- Dislocations
    Glenohumeral dislocation
    Acromioclavicular separation
    Sternoclavicular dislocation
- Fractures
    Clavicle fracture
    Acromial fracture
    Scapular fracture (body, neck, or glenoid)
    Proximal humerus fracture
- Other
    Rotator cuff tear
    Proximal biceps tendon rupture
    Pectoralis tendon rupture
    Scapulothoracic dissociation

■ BEDSIDE

Vital Signs

A complete set of vital signs is essential in any patient who has sustained a high-energy mechanism of injury or who has multiple injuries. In general, injury to the shoulder should not compromise the vital signs. As with trauma to other regions of the body, however, it should be expected that pain and anxiety will elevate the heart rate and blood pressure. The blood pressure should not be checked in the affected upper extremity because of patient discomfort. It is helpful to check the radial pulse in the affected arm while obtaining the pulse rate.

Selective History

How exactly was the shoulder injured?

Once the preliminary assessment has been completed and hemodynamic stability has been assured, a more detailed assessment of the mechanism of injury should be undertaken. In many cases an understanding of how the injury occurred can lead to an anatomic diagnosis. For example, Was the arm extended overhead (a position predisposing to anterior glenohumeral dislocation)? Did the patient receive a direct blow to the superior portion of the shoulder (the mechanism for acromioclavicular separation)? Did the patient sustain impact to or fall on an outstretched upper extremity (a mechanism for proximal humerus fracture)?

Can the patient localize the pain?

The examiner also should attempt to elicit from the patient the precise location of the pain. This will assist in narrowing the differential diagnosis and in focusing the subsequent physical and radiographic examinations. For example, patients with a fractured clavicle characteristically will note pain localized to the fracture site. In contrast, patients sustaining trapezius strain injury will note diffuse, poorly localized symptoms.

What are the patient-specific factors?

A final category of information that must be elicited during this portion of the evaluation includes factors specific to the individual patient. It is important to determine the age of the patient, as people are susceptible to different injury patterns about the shoulder at different ages. Elderly patients with age-related osteopenic bone are prone to fractures of the proximal humerus as a result of low-energy trauma. Similarly, older patients are more likely to sustain traumatic rotator cuff tear or biceps tendon rupture because of degeneration in these structures with aging. Another important piece of information to be obtained is any history of previous injury to the shoulder. This can be especially helpful in the evaluation of the young patient with a glenohumeral dislocation because of the high incidence of recurrent dislocations in this age group. Finally, as with all traumatic injuries, the patient must be questioned for the presence of any preexisting illnesses or chronic medical conditions that could affect the treatment of or the rehabilitation from the injury.

Selective Physical Examination

Inspection

The patient should be examined while disrobed from the waist up. Often much information regarding the severity of the injury can be obtained by noting how reluctant or willing the patient is to use the involved extremity to assist with disrobing and positioning. Notation should be made of any deformity, swelling, or asymmetry relative to the contralateral shoulder. Alteration of the bone or soft tissue contours may be indicative of glenohumeral dislocation. Prominence of the distal clavicle usually is due to acromioclavicular separation. A localized area of swelling often is associated with underlying fracture or joint dislocation. Any disruption in skin integrity must be identified and communication with underlying fracture or joint surfaces ruled out.

Palpation

The shoulder must be palpated systematically. A useful rule of thumb is to reserve palpation of the suspected area of injury for last. The examiner should develop a protocol for the examination so that the entire region can be evaluated fluidly and expeditiously. One possible protocol is to start anteriorly and medially at the sternoclavicular joint and then proceed laterally and posteriorly. Following palpation of the sternoclavicular joint, the clavicle can be palpated along its entire length along with the adjacent trapezius muscle. The acromioclavicular joint, acromion, and subacromial space are palpated next. Posterior examination then proceeds with palpation of the scapular spine and medial border. All areas of tenderness should be noted and an attempt made to correlate them with underlying anatomic structures.

Movements

An attempt should be made to gently move the glenohumeral joint. Significant pain with this maneuver and limitation of movement are signs of musculoskeletal injury. The range of motion allowed can be helpful in determining both the location and the type of injury present. Patients with fractures about the shoulder will tolerate little motion. Glenohumeral dislocation will limit internal and external rotation significantly. On the other hand, patients with acromioclavicular separation and sternoclavicular dislocation can have near normal, although painful, glenohumeral motion.

Special Tests

In addition to observation, palpation, and assessment of range of motion, a complete examination of the shoulder following injury requires special tests for determination of shoulder instability or musculotendinous disruption.

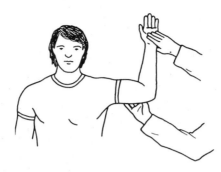

Figure 22–2 □ The apprehension sign for assessment of anterior shoulder instability. (From Birnbaum JS: The Musculoskeletal Manual, 2nd ed. Philadelphia, WB Saunders, 1986, p 64.)

Apprehension Sign (Fig. 22–2). This maneuver is indicated in the evaluation of the shoulder for potential anterior instability, which commonly occurs following anterior dislocation of the glenohumeral joint. The shoulder is gently rotated externally while being maintained in 90 degrees of abduction. Patients with instability will experience significant pain or "apprehension" with this maneuver because of anterior subluxation of the humerus.

Tests for Rotator Cuff Tear. Rotator cuff integrity may be specifically evaluated by testing the muscular functions of the cuff. The principal sign of a rotator cuff tear is weakness of external rotation (infraspinatus, teres minor) or midarc abduction (supraspinatus). The *drop arm sign* is also useful in the diagnosis of cuff tears. This test is performed by passively abducting the shoulder and asking the patient to actively maintain the abduction after the arm is released. Patients with rotator cuff tears will be unable to maintain midarc abduction.

Other Tests. If proximal biceps tendon rupture is suspected, the patient should be asked to actively flex the elbow against resistance. Patients with proximal tendon rupture will exhibit distal displacement of the biceps muscle mass and some weakness of biceps function relative to the contralateral upper extremity. If rupture of the pectoralis tendon is suspected, the patient should be asked to adduct the shoulder against resistance. Significant pain and weakness with this maneuver are signs of musculotendinous injury.

Neurovascular Examination

Because of the possibility of brachial plexus injury in association with shoulder trauma, a complete neurologic assessment of the affected upper extremity is indicated. This should include evaluation of reflex, sensory, and motor function. Certain simple tests can be performed to evaluate peripheral nerve function in the involved extremity. Abnormality of any one of the following tests warrants a more detailed examination:

Musculocutaneous nerve
  Motor: biceps (elbow flexion)
  Sensory: lateral aspect of proximal forearm
Axillary nerve
  Motor: deltoid (shoulder abduction)
  Sensory: lateral aspect of shoulder
Radial nerve
  Motor: wrist extension
  Sensory: dorsal thumb web space
Median nerve
  Motor: thumb interphalangeal joint flexion
  Sensory: radial three digits
Ulnar nerve
  Motor: first dorsal interosseous (index finger abduction)
  Sensory: small finger

The rare possibility of vascular injury in association with shoulder trauma must be ruled out also. Usually this can be done quickly by palpation of the radial and ulnar pulses at the wrist.

■ FURTHER ORDERS

All patients with shoulder pain following injury should be referred for radiographs of the shoulder. The standard screening views for the shoulder are AP views in both internal and external rotation, as well as an axillary lateral. Most fractures and dislocations of the shoulder can be diagnosed with these three views alone. If glenohumeral dislocation or scapular fracture is suspected, a scapular Y view also is often helpful. If clavicle fracture or sternoclavicular dislocation is suspected, a chest film is indicated.

■ MANAGEMENT

The immediate management of injuries to the shoulder region involves immobilization of the shoulder in a sling. This simple measure can improve patient comfort significantly. Immediate orthopaedic consultation is indicated for all fractures and dislocations about the shoulder. Many injuries to the shoulder are best managed nonoperatively. Certain traumatic conditions about the shoulder, such as proximal humerus fracture and rotator cuff tear, may require operative intervention however. This determination is made by the treating orthopaedist considering not only the injury but also important patient factors such as age and overall health.

With the exception of glenohumeral dislocation, open fractures, and the rare condition of scapulothoracic dissociation, all injuries to the shoulder can be treated definitively on a semielective basis.

The consulting orthopaedic surgeon occasionally may request additional radiographic studies in the evaluation of certain injuries about the shoulder girdle. One example of this is fracture of the scapular body or neck, in which case a CT scan may be necessary to rule out intraarticular penetration and displacement. Similarly an ultrasound examination may be requested to evaluate the integrity of the rotator cuff.

Glenohumeral dislocations are among the most common injuries to the musculoskeletal system. Most of these dislocations involve anterior displacement of the humeral head from the glenoid (Fig. 22–3). Glenohumeral dislocations must be reduced in a timely

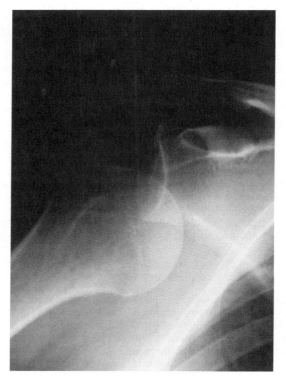

Figure 22–3 □ Classic radiographic appearance of anterior shoulder dislocation, with anterior and inferior displacement of the humeral head. An axillary lateral radiograph is necessary to confirm the anterior displacement.

manner to optimize outcome. The reduction commonly is performed in the emergency department using intravenous sedation or intraarticular injection of local anesthetic solution or both. AP and axillary lateral radiographs should be obtained following manipulation to document reduction of the joint. The shoulder then is placed in an immobilizer (sling and swathe). Young patients should be counseled extensively regarding the high incidence of recurrent dislocation.

Dislocations or separations of the acromioclavicular and sternoclavicular joints most commonly are managed nonoperatively. Patients are treated symptomatically with a brief period of shoulder immobilization followed by early institution of range of motion exercises. Occasionally, severe acromioclavicular separations may require operative intervention.

Fractures of the proximal humerus are problematic injuries for patients and orthopaedists alike. These injuries occur commonly in elderly patients with osteopenic bone. The fracture characteristically occurs at the surgical neck of the humerus with resulting impaction of the fracture fragments. Many of these fractures are best managed conservatively with a brief period of immobilization followed by controlled motion exercises. If the fracture is displaced significantly and the patient is relatively "high demand," prosthetic replacement of the humerus (hemiarthroplasty) may be indicated. In younger patients the treatment of proximal humerus fractures is somewhat controversial. Most orthopaedists agree that operative intervention is indicated for displaced fractures; however, considerable debate exists regarding the optimum method of fixation. Loss of motion is common following these fractures.

In contrast to fractures of the proximal humerus, fractures of the clavicle, acromion, and scapula rarely require operative intervention. Clavicle fractures may be managed initially in either a figure-8 orthosis or a simple shoulder sling. The results following treatment with both these devices appear to be equivalent; however, patients appear to tolerate the simple shoulder sling better. Acromial and scapular fractures most often are managed with a brief period of immobilization with a simple sling. With all fractures of the shoulder girdle, early controlled motion is essential and should be initiated as soon as patient comfort allows.

If there is an open fracture of the shoulder region, urgent orthopaedic intervention is indicated because of the significantly increased risk of infection. Patients with open fractures will require emergent operative debridement in addition to appropriate skeletal stabilization. Any open wounds should be covered with a sterile povidone-iodine (Betadine)-soaked gauze dressing pending definitive operative management.

Scapulothoracic dissociation involves complete dislocation of the scapula from the thoracic cage. This rare injury occurs following high-energy trauma and is characteristically associated with complex multisystem trauma. Major neurovascular disruptions are common.

In the absence of fracture or dislocation, injuries to the shoulder include muscle strain, rotator cuff tears, and muscle-tendon disruptions. These injuries should be treated much the same way as nontraumatic shoulder pain is. This treatment generally includes NSAIDs and physical therapy for shoulder range of motion and strengthening exercises. Steroid injections are not indicated for the treatment of shoulder trauma. Patients should be counseled that a protracted course is to be expected with slow resolution of pain and stiffness. In addition, certain patients with rotator cuff tears or proximal tendon ruptures may require surgical intervention following a trial of physical therapy.

23

ARM AND ELBOW PAIN

C. Michael LeCroy

The arm is defined by convention as the portion of the upper limb between the shoulder and elbow joints. Complaints of pain in the arm are rare in the absence of trauma. Elbow pain, on the other hand, can be encountered in a variety of traumatic and nontraumatic conditions. In most circumstances, injury to the arm and elbow occurs as a result of blunt, relatively high energy trauma. The injury to the arm or elbow may be an isolated injury, or it may be associated with multisystem trauma. Generally, the prognosis for injury to the arm is good; however, elbow injuries can result in chronic pain and stiffness in the absence of early and aggressive treatment. Like the shoulder, the elbow joint poorly tolerates prolonged immobilization.

■ PHONE CALL

Questions

1. **How was the arm or elbow injured?**
   An understanding of the mechanism of injury is critical in the evaluation of musculoskeletal trauma. This is the first step in the formulation of a differential diagnosis.
2. **Can the patient localize the pain to the arm or elbow?**
   The ability of the patient to localize the pain to a specific region of the arm or elbow can be very helpful in establishing a diagnosis.
3. **Is there gross deformity?**
   Obvious deformity of the arm or elbow usually indicates fracture or dislocation or both.
4. **Is there an associated skin wound or laceration?**
   An open wound should alert the physician to the potential for an open fracture or intraarticular communication. These conditions require urgent evaluation and treatment.
5. **Can the patient move the extremity spontaneously?**
   Spontaneous or voluntary movements of the extremity distal to the site of injury can provide a rough assessment of whether there is concomitant neurologic injury. This must be evaluated subsequently by physical examination.
6. **Are there any additional injuries?**
   As with all trauma to the musculoskeletal system, associ-

ated injuries to the musculoskeletal system as well as to other body systems must be excluded. This is particularly important in cases of high-energy trauma, in which the incidence of associated injuries is high.

7. Is the patient hemodynamically stable?

Hemodynamic stability is the first priority of management in all trauma victims. If the patient is not hemodynamically stable, attention should be turned to the ABCs (airway, breathing, circulation) before the musculoskeletal injury is evaluated.

Orders

1. To provide the patient as much pain relief as possible and to prevent further damage, ask the RN to immobilize the elbow. This can be accomplished easily using an arm sling or even by simply resting the affected arm on a pillow with the elbow slightly flexed.
2. If the patient has sustained a high-energy mechanism of injury, such as a motor vehicle accident, ask the RN to obtain immediate consultation with a general trauma specialist (emergency medicine physician or general surgeon).

Inform RN

"I will arrive at the bedside/emergency department within 30 minutes."

In the absence of other organ system injuries, injury to the arm and elbow is seldom life or limb threatening. If an open fracture or elbow dislocation is suspected from the described injury mechanism and history, the patient should be evaluated on an urgent basis. In general, to optimize outcome and minimize patient discomfort, all injuries to the arm and elbow should be evaluated as soon as possible.

■ ELEVATOR THOUGHTS

- Strains
    None
- Sprains
    Ulnar collateral ligament injury (elbow)
    Radial collateral ligament injury (elbow)
- Dislocations
    Ulnohumeral dislocation (elbow dislocation)
    Radial head dislocation
- Fractures
    Humeral shaft fracture

Distal humerus fracture (supracondylar vs. intercondylar)
Olecranon fracture
Coronoid process fracture
Radial head fracture
- Other
   Distal biceps tendon rupture

■ BEDSIDE

Vital Signs

A complete set of vital signs is essential in any patient who has sustained a high-energy trauma. In general, injury to the arm or elbow should not compromise the vital signs. As with trauma to other regions of the body, it should be expected that pain and anxiety will elevate the blood pressure and heart rate. The blood pressure should not be checked in the injured arm because of patient discomfort. It is helpful to check the radial pulse in the affected arm, however, to ensure vascular integrity of the extremity.

Selective History

How exactly was the arm or elbow injured?

Once the preliminary assessment is completed and hemodynamic stability has been assured, attention can be turned to a more detailed assessment of the mechanism of injury. Often an understanding of how the injury occurred can lead to an anatomic diagnosis. For example, Did the patient sustain a direct blow to the arm (a common mechanism for fractures of the humerus and elbow region), or did the patient fall onto an outstretched extremity (a common mechanism for elbow dislocation)? Is the injury a result of a twisting force to the elbow (collateral ligament injury)? Did the patient feel or hear a "pop" in the elbow region (biceps tendon rupture)?

Can the patient localize the pain?

The patient should be asked if he or she can localize the pain. Not infrequently, injuries to the shoulder region present with lateral arm pain. Thus arm pain may be confused with pain originating in the shoulder. It is also helpful to have the patient localize any elbow pain to the medial, lateral, posterior, or anterior aspects of the joint. This information will assist the examiner in establishing the diagnosis, as well as in focusing the physical and radiographic examinations.

What are the patient-specific factors?

Specific patient factors are important to consider in the evaluation of the patient with injury to the arm or elbow. These include the patient's age and dominant upper extremity. Older patients are susceptible to bone and soft tissue injuries from low-energy trauma. The handedness (i.e., right vs. left) of the patient is an important consideration in the formulation of a treatment plan and prognosis for injuries to the upper extremity. Injuries to the dominant upper extremity can be expected to cause more functional difficulties for the patient. Any history of previous injury to the arm or elbow should also be elicited. Finally, patients must be questioned carefully for any preexisting illnesses or chronic medical conditions that could affect the treatment of or the rehabilitation from the injury.

Selective Physical Examination

Inspection

The entire length of both upper extremities should be exposed for visual inspection. The injured arm and elbow should be carefully examined for deformity or swelling, which may indicate a fracture or dislocation. Deformity or swelling often can be best appreciated by comparison to the contralateral uninjured upper extremity. With humeral fractures the arm may appear shortened or angulated. With elbow dislocation, disruption of the normal contours of the elbow is often obvious. The arm and elbow also must be inspected carefully for any disruption of skin integrity. The communication of any wounds or lacerations with underlying fracture or articular surfaces must be ruled out.

Palpation

The arm and elbow should be palpated systematically. It is important to palpate all aspects of the elbow, as injury in a variety of anatomic locations can present with "elbow pain." The condyles and epicondyles of the distal humerus should be palpated medially and laterally, along with the olecranon posteriorly. The radial and ulnar collateral ligaments of the elbow also should be palpated. With fractures of the arm and elbow, movement of the fracture surfaces or crepitation often can be appreciated with gentle palpation. All areas of localized tenderness and swelling should be noted and an attempt made to correlate them with underlying anatomic structures.

Movements

An attempt should be made to gently move the elbow joint. Appreciable pain or limitation of motion with this maneuver is a sign of significant musculoskeletal injury. The range of motion allowed by the patient can be helpful in determining both the location and type of injury. Patients with elbow dislocation will have markedly restricted motion. Conversely, a near normal range of motion often can rule out any significant fracture or dislocation about the arm or elbow.

Special Tests

In addition to observation, palpation, and assessment of range of motion, a complete examination of the arm and elbow following trauma requires special tests for determination of elbow instability or musculotendinous disruption.

Elbow Instability Test. The integrity of the collateral ligaments of the elbow may be evaluated by sequentially applying varus and valgus stresses to the elbow with the joint gently flexed 20 to 30 degrees. The upper hand of the examiner is used to stabilize the arm, and the lower hand is used to apply a varus stress (for evaluation of the radial collateral ligament) and a valgus stress (for evaluation of the ulnar collateral ligament). Collateral ligament injury is noted with excessive opening of the elbow joint to either or both of these stresses. This maneuver also should be performed on the contralateral uninjured elbow to allow appreciation of subtle differences.

Tests for Distal Biceps Tendon Rupture. Patients with distal biceps tendon rupture will exhibit significant tenderness to palpation of the distal arm and elbow anteriorly. In addition, the patient should be asked to actively flex the elbow against resistance. Proximal displacement of the biceps muscle mass and weakness of elbow flexion relative to the contralateral upper extremity will indicate distal tendon rupture.

Neurovascular Examination

A focused neurologic assessment of the injured extremity is necessary because of the relatively high incidence of neurologic injury with fractures and dislocations of the arm and elbow. Fractures of the humeral shaft often are associated with radial nerve injury. Any fracture or dislocation about the elbow may damage the ulnar nerve because of its relatively subcutaneous position behind the medial epicondyle. Likewise, the median nerve may be injured with posterior ulnohumeral dislocation. Thus it is critical to assess the integrity of motor and sensory function of all three nerves in the forearm, wrist, and hand. The tests described in Chapter 22 for quick assessment of peripheral nerve function in the upper extremity should be performed. Occasionally the brachial artery also will be injured with arm or elbow trauma. Palpation of the radial and ulnar pulses at the wrist can verify the integrity of vascular function.

■ FURTHER ORDERS

All patients sustaining arm or elbow trauma should be referred for radiographs of the humerus or elbow. If the patient's pain cannot be localized reliably, it is useful to image both the humerus and the elbow. This will allow evaluation of the entire humerus, including the glenohumeral articulation, the elbow joint, and the proximal forearm. Standard screening radiographs for both the humerus and the elbow consist simply of AP and lateral views. With fracture or dislocation, it often is not possible to position the extremity adequately for images in the true coronal and sagittal planes; nevertheless, an attempt should be made to obtain two orthogonal images.

■ MANAGEMENT

The immediate management of trauma to the arm and elbow requires immobilization of the extremity to minimize discomfort and prevent further soft tissue trauma. The most effective way to immobilize the elbow is to apply a simple posterior long arm plaster splint. If fracture of the humerus is suspected or identified, a coaptation plaster splint provides the most effective immobilization. If plaster splints are not available, a shoulder sling and swathe can be used; however, less effective pain relief and immobilization should be anticipated.

Immediate orthopaedic consultation is indicated for all fractures and dislocations of the humerus and elbow. Dislocations of the ul-

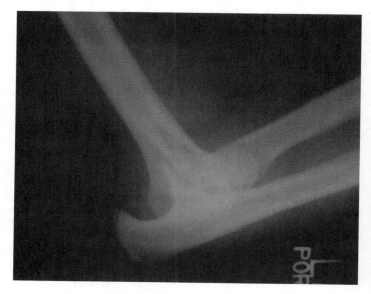

Figure 23–1 □ Posterior elbow dislocation with complete displacement of the ulnohumeral articulation.

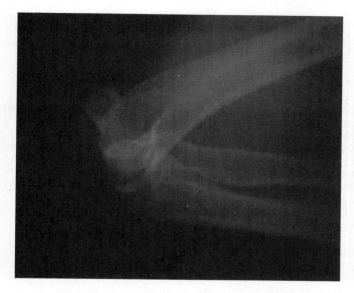

Figure 23–2 □ Complex fracture of the olecranon.

nohumeral joint or the radial head require urgent reduction to maximize potential for return of function (Fig. 23–1). The reduction commonly is performed in the emergency department using intravenous sedation or intraarticular injection of local anesthetic solution. The elbow most commonly is splinted for a brief period following reduction. Early, controlled range of motion is indicated to prevent stiffness. The physician also should remember that dislocations about the elbow commonly are associated with fractures of either the distal humerus (ulnohumeral dislocation) or forearm (radial head dislocation).

Most fractures of the humeral shaft are managed effectively nonoperatively, and a good prognosis is expected. The arm usually is placed into a fracture brace once the acute swelling has subsided. This functional brace allows full mobilization of the shoulder and elbow joints proximal and distal to the fracture. In contrast, displaced fractures of the distal humerus and olecranon in adults most commonly are treated with operative reduction and fixation (Fig. 23–2). An attempt should be made to anatomically reduce any intraarticular extension of the fracture and to obtain stable fixation that will allow early motion of the elbow joint.

Fractures of the radial head and coronoid process may require surgery, depending on the amount of displacement, the size of the fracture fragments, and individual patient considerations. All decisions regarding surgical treatment should be made by the treating orthopaedist with consideration given to the patient's age, overall health, and handedness. If skin integrity is not disrupted (i.e., open fracture), most fractures of the arm and elbow can be managed definitively on a semielective basis.

Open fractures require emergent orthopaedic intervention because of the significantly increased risk of infection. Patients with open fractures will require emergent operative debridement in addition to appropriate skeletal stabilization. Any open wounds should be covered with a sterile betadine-soaked gauze dressing pending definitive treatment.

Soft tissue trauma to the elbow region usually is managed nonoperatively. Patients with collateral ligament injuries should be treated with a brief period of immobilization followed by range of motion and strengthening exercises with physical therapy. Early active elbow motion is particularly important in the management of contusions to the distal arm and elbow to reduce the potential for posttraumatic heterotopic ossification. NSAIDs are also helpful in the treatment of soft tissue trauma to the arm and elbow. Rupture of the distal biceps tendon in young adult patients is managed most effectively with operative repair because of the significant reduction in elbow flexion strength without repair.

As with other types of musculoskeletal trauma, cold therapy, compression, and extremity elevation are also useful in the acute management of bone or soft tissue trauma to the arm and elbow.

24

FOREARM AND WRIST PAIN

C. Michael LeCroy

Injuries to the forearm and wrist are common musculoskeletal conditions in adults. The usual mechanism of injury is a fall onto the outstretched extremity; however, direct blunt trauma to this region also occurs. Fractures and dislocations in the forearm and wrist often are seen in association with other musculoskeletal injuries in victims of high-energy trauma. Although the prognosis for injuries to the forearm generally is good, fractures and dislocations of the wrist can have significant long term sequelae. For the purposes of this text, the *wrist* will be defined as including the distal radius and ulna as well as the eight carpal bones.

■ PHONE CALL

Questions

1. **How was the forearm or wrist injured?**

   An understanding of the mechanism of injury is critical in the evaluation of musculoskeletal trauma. This is the first step in the formulation of a differential diagnosis.

2. **Is the pain localized to the forearm or to the wrist?**

   The ability of the patient to localize the pain to a specific region of the forearm or wrist can be very helpful in establishing a diagnosis.

3. **Is there gross deformity?**

   Obvious deformity of the forearm or wrist usually indicates fracture or dislocation or both.

4. **Is there an associated skin wound or laceration?**

   An open wound should alert the physician to the potential for an open fracture or intraarticular communication. These conditions require urgent evaluation and treatment.

5. **Can the patient move his fingers?**

   Spontaneous or voluntary movements of the extremity distal to the site of injury can provide a rough assessment of whether there is concomitant neurologic injury. This must be evaluated subsequently by physical examination.

6. **Are there any additional injuries?**

   As with all trauma to the musculoskeletal system, associated injuries to the musculoskeletal system as well as to other body systems must be excluded. This is particularly important in cases of high-energy trauma, in which the incidence of associated injuries is high.

7. **Is the patient hemodynamically stable?**
   Hemodynamic stability is the first priority of management in all trauma victims. If the patient is not hemodynamically stable, attention should be turned to the ABCs (airway, breathing, circulation) before the musculoskeletal injury is evaluated.

Orders

1. Ask the RN to elevate and rest the injured extremity on a pillow or blanket. This will help immobilize the area of injury and provide partial pain relief. A plaster splint should not be applied until the extremity has been examined.
2. If the patient has sustained a high-energy mechanism of injury, such as a motor vehicle accident or fall from a height, ask the RN to obtain immediate consultation with a general trauma specialist (emergency medicine physician or general surgeon).

Inform RN

"I will arrive at the bedside within 30 minutes."

In the absence of other organ system injuries, trauma to the forearm and wrist rarely is life or limb threatening. The one exception to this is a compartment syndrome of the forearm, which should be suspected following a severe crushing injury. Failure to recognize and promptly treat a compartment syndrome can cause irreversible muscle necrosis and possibly compromise limb viability. Also, if an open fracture or dislocation is suspected, the patient should be evaluated as soon as possible. In general, to optimize outcome and minimize patient discomfort, all injuries to the forearm and wrist should be evaluated as soon as possible.

■ ELEVATOR THOUGHTS

- Strains
  - None
- Sprains
  - Triangular fibrocartilage complex injury (wrist sprain)
- Dislocations
  - Distal radioulnar joint dislocation
  - Radiocarpal dislocation
  - Lunate or perilunate dislocation
  - Scapholunate dissociation
- Fractures
  - Radial shaft fracture

Ulnar shaft fracture

Both-bones forearm fracture (fractures of the radial and ulnar shafts)

Distal radius fracture (with or without ulnar styloid fracture)

Scaphoid fracture

Other carpal bone fracture

- Other

Compartment syndrome of forearm

■ BEDSIDE

Vital Signs

A complete set of vital signs should be obtained in any patient who has sustained an injury. Trauma to the forearm and wrist generally will not cause abnormal vital signs; however, it should be anticipated that pain and anxiety will elevate the heart rate and blood pressure. The blood pressure should not be checked in the injured extremity because of patient discomfort. It is helpful to check the radial pulse in the affected arm to assess the vascular integrity of the extremity.

Selective History

How exactly was the forearm or wrist injured?

Following preliminary assessment of the patient, the mechanism of injury should be evaluated in as much detail as possible. As with trauma to other anatomic regions, an understanding of how the injury occurred can often alert the physician to certain types of injuries. For example, Did the patient sustain a direct blow to the forearm (radial or ulnar shaft fracture)? Did the patient fall onto an outstretched hand and wrist (distal radius fracture, carpal bone fracture or dislocation)? Was there a crushing injury to the forearm (compartment syndrome)?

Can the patient localize the pain?

The patient should be asked to localize the pain. Most patients with injury to the wrist region will localize their pain to this area. On the other hand, patients with forearm trauma often will have diffuse pain without localization. In addition, injuries to the elbow region may present with forearm pain.

What are the patient-specific factors?

During the initial evaluation the examiner also should consider several specific patient factors, including the patient's age, preexisting illnesses or comorbid factors, and the handedness (i.e., right vs. left) of the patient. Older patients with osteopenic bone are notoriously susceptible to fractures of the distal radius.

Likewise, certain preexisting illnesses or conditions such as diabetes, stroke, cardiac disease, or chronic corticosteroid use can affect the treatment and rehabilitation regimens. The patient should be asked if the forearm or wrist has been injured previously. Finally the dominant upper extremity always should be determined in injuries to the forearm and wrist. This information is important in formulating a treatment plan and in the prognosis for injuries to the upper extremity.

Selective Physical Examination

Inspection

The entire length of both upper extremities should be exposed for visual inspection. The injured forearm and wrist should be examined carefully for swelling or deformity. Because of the subcutaneous position of the bones and joints in this area of the body, most fractures and dislocations in this region will present with discernible deformities. These often can be best appreciated by comparing them to the uninjured contralateral upper extremity. The forearm and wrist also must be carefully assessed for any disruption of skin integrity. The communication of any wounds or lacerations with underlying fracture or joint surfaces must be ruled out.

Palpation

The forearm and wrist should be palpated systematically. In general, the area of pain localized by the patient (the suspected area of injury) should be palpated last. With fractures of the radius and ulna, movement of the fracture surfaces or crepitation often can be appreciated with gentle palpation. The wrist should be palpated for tenderness in the region of the anatomic snuffbox, which can indicate fracture of the scaphoid. All areas of tenderness and deformity should be noted and an attempt made to correlate these areas with underlying anatomic structures. Diffuse and marked swelling of the entire forearm in association with a crushing injury may herald a compartment syndrome.

Movements

The examiner should attempt to gently move the elbow and wrist joints. Significant pain or limitation of motion with this maneuver is a sign of musculoskeletal injury. The range of motion allowed by the patient can be helpful in determining the location, type, and severity of the injury. Patients with a dislocated wrist will permit little wrist motion. If motion of the wrist and elbow is normal or nearly so, passive supination and pronation of the forearm may help identify more subtle injury. If a compartment syndrome is suspected on the basis of the mechanism of injury and swelling, the wrist and hand should be evaluated for pain with passive stretch of the muscle-tendon units. This is the most sensitive test for compartment syndrome.

Neurovascular Examination

A focused neurologic assessment of the injured upper extremity is necessary with trauma to the forearm and wrist. A careful evaluation of peripheral nerve function distal to the area of injury should be attempted. This can be accomplished effectively using the following quick tests. Abnormal results in any one of the following tests warrants a more detailed examination:

Radial nerve
> *Motor:* thumb interphalangeal (IP) joint extension (posterior interosseous nerve)
> *Sensory:* dorsal thumb web space (superficial radial nerve)

Median nerve
> *Motor:* index finger proximal interphalangeal (PIP) joint flexion; thumb IP joint flexion (anterior interosseous nerve)
> *Sensory:* radial three digits (thumb, index, and long)

Ulnar nerve
> *Motor:* first dorsal interosseous (index finger abduction)
> *Sensory:* small finger

The adequacy of vascular perfusion of the limb also should be verified with any trauma to the forearm or wrist. The radial and ulnar pulses usually can be palpated at the wrist, even in the presence of swelling. Doppler evaluation occasionally may be necessary. Vascular function distal to the wrist level can be assessed through capillary refill time in each digit.

■ FURTHER ORDERS

All patients sustaining forearm or wrist trauma should be referred for radiographs. Standard screening radiographs for both the forearm and wrist consist of AP and lateral views. If there is fracture or dislocation, the patient often will not tolerate positioning of the extremity in the true coronal and sagittal planes; nevertheless, attempts should be made to obtain two images at perpendicular angles. If the patient's pain cannot be localized reliably and no deformity is immediately obvious, it is wise to obtain radiographs of both the forearm and wrist. Also, if fracture of the radial or ulnar shafts is suspected, images of both the wrist and elbow should be obtained because of the possibility of associated dislocation of the distal radioulnar joint (Galeazzi fracture) or proximal radioulnar joint (Monteggia fracture).

■ MANAGEMENT

The immediate management of trauma to the forearm and wrist requires immobilization of the extremity to minimize patient discomfort and to prevent further soft tissue trauma. The forearm and wrist are immobilized most effectively with a plaster sugar tong splint applied with the forearm in neutral pronation-supination. The forearm also should be elevated to minimize swelling. If plaster is not available, the extremity can be immobilized less effectively with an arm board strapped loosely to the forearm. Care should be taken to avoid excessive compression of the extremity, which might exacerbate swelling or potentially compromise vascular perfusion.

If radiographs do not disclose fracture and soft tissue trauma is suspected (e.g., wrist sprain), the patient should be treated symptomatically with a brief period of immobilization of the extremity, preferably with a removable orthosis. Range of motion exercises should be instituted once the acute swelling and tenderness have subsided. NSAIDs also are helpful in the acute stage.

Orthopaedic consultation is indicated for all fractures and dislocations of the forearm, wrist, and carpus. Immediate evaluation is necessary for dislocations of the radiocarpal joint or carpal bones, as urgent reduction is often necessary. These injuries frequently are associated with fractures of the distal radius or carpal bones. Although the reduction often may be obtained with closed techniques, most such injuries are unstable and require subsequent operative reconstruction.

Scapholunate dissociation involves dislocation of the scaphoid-lunate articulation in the proximal carpal row. The mechanism is disruption of the scapholunate interosseous ligaments. Scapholunate dissociations easily may be missed on initial evaluation, and many of these injuries erroneously are assumed to be simple wrist sprains. If not recognized and treated early, scapholunate dissociation can lead to significant long-term complications of wrist stiffness and pain. Radiographic criteria for diagnosis of scapholunate dissociation include widening of the scapholunate joint space on the AP image of the wrist and increase in the scapholunate angle on the lateral image. Scapholunate dissociation is best managed acutely with operative reduction and volar ligament repair.

Isolated fractures of the ulnar shaft commonly are managed nonoperatively with splint or cast immobilization, with generally good results expected. On the other hand, fractures of the shaft of the radius in adults are best managed with operative reduction and stabilization, particularly when such fractures are associated with dislocation of the distal radioulnar joint (Galeazzi fracture). Both-bones forearm fractures in skeletally mature patients should be treated with operative reduction and fixation (Fig. 24–1). In the absence of open fracture or neurovascular compromise, fractures of the forearm can be managed definitively on a semielective basis.

Fractures of the distal radius represent one of the most common injuries to the musculoskeletal system (Fig. 24–2). A bimodal distribution of these fractures is noted, with occurrence in older patients following low-energy trauma and occurrence in young adult patients following high-energy trauma. In older patients,

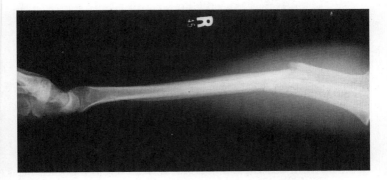

Figure 24–1 □ Lateral radiograph of the forearm demonstrating a proximal both-bones forearm fracture.

distal radius fractures most often are managed with closed reduction and splinting and local anesthesia in the emergency department or the office of the treating orthopaedic physician. During the reduction, emphasis is placed on restoring the length and distal angulation of the radius, as well as reducing any intraarticular extension. If an acceptable reduction is obtained, the patient's wrist commonly is placed into a cast, once the acute swelling has subsided, for 6 to 8 weeks. Many elderly patients will experience some settling of the fracture during closed treatment because of dorsal comminution and relative osteopenia. Nevertheless, good functional results can be expected in the elderly patient following most distal radius fractures.

In the young adult patient, distal radius fractures normally are the result of high-energy trauma. These fractures characteristically exhibit significant comminution and intraarticular extension. Although closed reduction may be attempted, many distal radius fractures in young patients are best managed with operative intervention using closed vs. open reduction and internal or external fixation techniques. Indications for operative intervention include articular surface displacement and instability due to significant comminution. With operative treatment, priority is given to restoration of radial length and reduction of the articular surface, with acceptable reduction requiring less than 2 mm displacement. As with forearm fractures, most distal radius fractures can be splinted acutely and treated definitively on a semielective basis. Although most distal radius fractures will heal uneventfully, the functional result is variable in young patients and depends on the reduction obtained. Long-term sequelae of wrist stiffness and weakened grip strength are not uncommon.

Fractures of the carpal bones usually are treated nonoperatively, generally with good outcomes. The one exception is fracture of the scaphoid (carpal navicular). Because of its tenuous blood supply, displaced fractures of the scaphoid are associated with a high incidence of nonunion and avascular necrosis (Fig. 24–3). For this reason, patients with significant wrist tenderness in the anatomic snuffbox, regardless of whether a fracture is seen on radiographs, should be managed acutely with immobilization of the wrist and thumb (thumb spica splint) and follow-up evaluation in 1 week. The evaluating orthopaedist may obtain additional radiographic views of the carpus to evaluate further for scaphoid fracture. Displaced fractures of the scaphoid require operative intervention in most cases.

If there is an open fracture or an intraarticular penetrating injury, immediate orthopaedic evaluation and treatment is indicated because of the high risk of infection. Such injuries most often will require urgent operative debridement or joint exploration and irri-

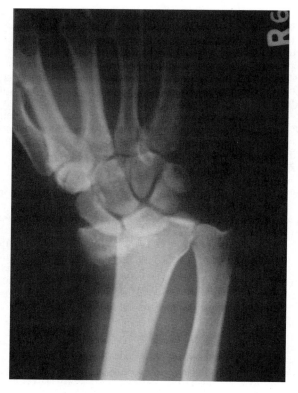

Figure 24–2 □ Fracture of the distal radius.

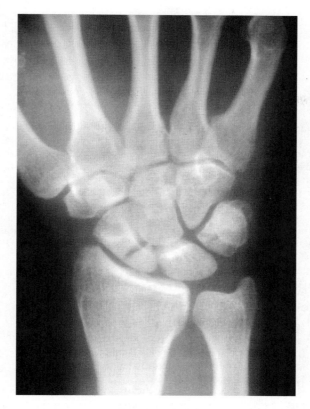

Figure 24–3 □ Displaced fracture of the scaphoid. This fracture is associated with a high incidence of nonunion and osteonecrosis.

gation. Any open fracture wounds should be covered with a sterile betadine-soaked gauze dressing pending definitive treatment.

If compartment syndrome is suspected on the basis of the history of injury and the physical examination, emergent orthopaedic consultation is indicated. The forearm is second only to the leg in the incidence of compartment syndrome. A compartment syndrome must be treated with emergent fasciotomy. Compartment syndromes are discussed in more detail in Chapter 32.

25

HAND PAIN

C. Michael LeCroy

Injury to the hand is one of the most common musculoskeletal conditions presenting for emergency department evaluation. Characteristically, most hand trauma occurs as an isolated injury. A variety of mechanisms may be responsible, including industrial accidents, recreational injuries, and blunt trauma. In contrast to other types of extremity trauma, most hand injuries involve lacerations or wounds with associated soft tissue trauma. In most cases, early, aggressive treatment is necessary to ensure optimal recovery of function. For the purposes of this text, the hand will be defined as the structures distal to the carpometacarpal joints.

■ PHONE CALL

Questions

1. **How was the hand injured?**
   An understanding of the mechanism of injury is critical in the evaluation of musculoskeletal trauma. This is the first step in the formulation of a differential diagnosis.
2. **Is there an associated skin wound or laceration?**
   An open wound on the hand should alert the physician to the potential for an open fracture, intraarticular communication, tendon laceration, or neurovascular injury. These conditions require urgent evaluation and treatment.
3. **Is there a complete or near complete digital amputation?**
   These injuries should alert the physician to the likelihood of significant bone and soft tissue trauma to the hand. High-energy crushing and mangling mechanisms normally are responsible. Urgent evaluation is necessary to assess viability of the amputated digit(s).
4. **Is there gross deformity or swelling?**
   Obvious deformity or swelling of the hand usually indicates fracture or dislocation or both.
5. **Can the patient localize the pain to a specific area?**
   The ability of the patient to localize the pain to a specific region of the hand can be helpful in establishing a diagnosis.
6. **Can the patient move all his fingers?**
   Spontaneous or voluntary movements of the fingers can provide a rough assessment of whether there is concomitant

neurologic injury or tendon lacerations. This must be evaluated subsequently by physical examination.

7. **Are there any additional injuries?**

As with all trauma to the musculoskeletal system, associated injuries to other body systems must be ruled out. This is particularly important in cases of high-energy trauma, in which the incidence of associated injuries is high.

8. **Is the patient hemodynamically stable?**

Hemodynamic stability is the first priority of management in all trauma victims. If the patient is not hemodynamically stable, attention should be turned to the ABCs (airway, breathing, circulation) before the musculoskeletal injury is evaluated.

Orders

1. Ask the RN to elevate and rest the injured hand on a pillow or blanket to relatively immobilize the injured area and provide partial pain relief.
2. If there is a skin laceration with significant bleeding, ask the RN to apply a sterile compressive dressing to the hand.
3. If the patient has sustained an amputation, ask the RN to wrap the amputated part (if available) in gauze, place it in a plastic bag filled with saline, and then place the bag into ice. Ice should never be applied directly to the amputated part, as it will cause thermal damage, which may prohibit attempted replantation of the digit.
4. If the patient has sustained a high-energy mechanism of injury, such as a motor vehicle accident, ask the RN to obtain immediate consultation with a general trauma specialist (emergency medicine physician or general surgeon).

Inform RN

"I will arrive at the bedside within 30 minutes."

In the absence of other organ system injuries, injury to the hand is rarely life or limb threatening. However, lacerations and amputations in the hand can be associated with significant blood loss and should be evaluated as soon as possible, particularly if replantation is to be considered. Suspected compartment syndrome in the hand following a crushing injury also must be evaluated and treated urgently to prevent irreversible muscle necrosis and compromised limb function. Similarly, a history of high-pressure injection injury or thermal injury to the hand should be evaluated urgently. As in other extremity injuries, suspected open fractures, intraarticular injuries, and dislocations should be evaluated in timely fashion. In general, to optimize outcome and minimize patient discomfort, all injuries to the hand should be evaluated on an urgent basis.

■ ELEVATOR THOUGHTS

- Strains
    None
- Sprains
    Jammed finger (digital collateral ligament injury)
    Gamekeeper's thumb (ulnar collateral ligament injury)
- Dislocations
    Carpometacarpal dislocation
    Metacarpophalangeal dislocation
    Interphalangeal dislocation
- Fractures
    Metacarpal shaft fracture
    Metacarpal neck fracture
    Phalangeal fracture
    Tuft fracture (tip of distal phalanx)
- Other
    Compartment syndrome of hand
    Amputation or near amputation
    High-pressure injection injury
    Thermal injury (burn, chemical burn, electrical injury, cold
        injury)
    Nailbed injury
    Flexor tendon injury
    Extensor tendon injury

■ BEDSIDE

Vital Signs

A complete set of vital signs should be obtained in all trauma
victims. Hand injuries usually will not compromise the vital signs.
Hand lacerations, however, can be associated with significant
bleeding and subsequent tachycardia. Also, it should be expected
that the pain and anxiety accompanying hand injuries will increase
the pulse rate and blood pressure. The blood pressure should not
be checked in the injured extremity because of patient discomfort.

Selective History

How exactly was the hand injured?
    Once the initial assessment is completed, a more thorough in-
vestigation into the precise mechanism of injury is indicated. An
understanding of how the injury occurred can often alert the examiner to certain types of injuries. For example, patients who
strike a fixed object with a clenched fist frequently fracture the
small finger metacarpal neck (boxer's fracture). Similarly an abduction force to the base of the thumb is likely to produce an

ulnar collateral ligament injury (gamekeeper's thumb). Patients with deep lacerations to the volar aspect of the hand or digits are at risk for flexor tendon or neurovascular injury. A compartment syndrome may develop subsequent to a crushing injury to the hand.

Is there a history of high-pressure injection or thermal injury to the hand?

Injection of toxic substances such as paints, sealants, or lubricants into a digit or hand should alert the examiner to the potential for serious injury. Similarly a history of thermal injury (burns, chemical burns, electrical injury, cold injury) necessitates urgent evaluation and treatment. It should be remembered that these injuries initially may have a benign appearance but rapidly lead to tissue destruction if left untreated.

Can the patient localize the pain?

The patient should be asked if he can localize the pain. This is often difficult, as injury anywhere in the hand may present with diffuse pain and swelling. If signs of injury are obvious, such as skin laceration or deformity, localization of symptoms may be unnecessary. In more subtle trauma to the hand, however, every effort should be made to have the patient indicate the painful site as precisely as possible.

What are the patient-specific factors?

With injury to the hand, factors specific to the individual patient are critical in determining the course of treatment and prognosis. These factors, which should be elicited during the initial evaluation, include the patient's age, the patient's handedness (i.e., right vs. left), the patient's occupation, and any comorbid conditions. All these factors must be taken into consideration by the treating physician in determining the best course of treatment. In general the treatment will be more aggressive for injuries to the dominant hand and for injuries in patients for whom the functional demands of the hand are high. Certain factors, such as advanced age or history of cigarette smoking, may be seen as contraindications to replantation of a severed digit.

Selective Physical Examination

Inspection

All clothing and jewelry should be removed to allow complete visual inspection of the entire hand. Most fractures and dislocations in the hand are heralded by deformity and swelling. These findings often can be best appreciated by a comparison to the contralateral uninjured hand. The resting position, or attitude, of the digits also should be noted. Flexor tendon lacerations will result in extension of the involved digit(s), whereas extensor tendon injuries result in flexion. All digits should be inspected carefully for rotational deformity, which can occur with phalangeal or metacarpal fractures. The rotation of the digits is best assessed by having the patient flex the fingers into a fist.

Since most hand trauma is associated with open skin wounds, great care should be taken to identify all areas of disrupted skin integrity. Active bleeding should be noted. The condition of the nailbed on the injured digit should be assessed. Communication of any wounds or lacerations with underlying fracture or joint surfaces must be ascertained. Finally, pinpoint injection sites or tissue destruction due to thermal injury should be noted.

Palpation

The entire hand should be palpated systematically from the carpometacarpal joints to the tips of the fingers. Generally the suspected area of injury should be palpated last. Because of the subcutaneous position of the bones and joints in the hand, movement of fracture surfaces or crepitation usually can be appreciated with gentle palpation. All areas of tenderness should be noted and an attempt made to correlate these areas with the underlying anatomic structures. Diffuse and marked swelling of the entire hand following a crushing injury may indicate a developing compartment syndrome.

Movements

In the absence of obvious bone deformity or skin laceration, an attempt should be made to gently range the carpometacarpal, metacarpophalangeal, and interphalangeal joints of the hand. Appreciable pain or limitation of motion is a sign of significant musculoskeletal injury. With all injuries to the hand, active range of motion of the digits also should be assessed. Any limitation of motion should be noted. Inability to move the fingers can have various causes. These are addressed separately in Chapter 26. If compartment syndrome of the hand is suspected on the basis of the mechanism of injury and swelling, the hand should be evaluated for pain with passive stretch of the muscle-tendon units. This can be accomplished simply by passive flexion and extension of the digits. Pain with passive stretch is the most sensitive test for compartment syndrome.

Neurovascular Examination

Injuries at the level of the hand usually will not involve trauma to major peripheral nerves. The digital nerves often are affected, however, and the status of digital nerve function should be assessed on the radial and ulnar aspects of each injured digit. Two-point discrimination on the tip of the finger is a useful screening tool; however, subtle digital nerve injury may be missed if sensation is not checked on the radial and ulnar aspects of each fingertip. It should also be remembered that sensation in the fingertips is a combination of median (thumb, index, long, and radial aspect of ring) and ulnar (ulnar aspect of ring and small) nerve functions.

Vascular injury also is quite common with trauma to the hand. The hand and digits have a rich collateral circulation and generally can tolerate isolated vascular disruptions. The viability of vascular flow to each injured digit should be carefully evaluated. The digit can be inspected for evidence of pallor or loss of skin turgor. The digit also should be evaluated for capillary refill time at the fingertip. Normal capillary refill time is less than 3 seconds.

■ FURTHER ORDERS

All patients sustaining an injury to the hand should be sent for plain radiographs of the hand. The standard radiographic views for the hand are AP, lateral, and oblique. The oblique image is necessary because of the inevitable overlapping of the metacarpals and phalanges on the lateral view. If phalangeal injury is suspected, the patient must be urged to hold the digit fully extended to allow complete visualization of the interphalangeal joints.

■ MANAGEMENT

The immediate management of trauma to the hand requires immobilization to minimize patient discomfort and to prevent further soft tissue damage. The hand can be effectively immobilized with a plaster splint or arm board extending along either the volar or dorsal aspect of the hand to the forearm. The hand should be elevated following immobilization to minimize swelling. Care should be taken to avoid excessive compression of the hand, which might potentially compromise the vascular perfusion.

Significant bleeding from lacerations to the hand should be controlled as soon as possible. This almost always can be accomplished with a compressive gauze dressing and elevation of the hand above heart level. If significant bleeding persists with these measures, direct manual pressure should be applied to the area of injury. The temptation to blindly clamp small blood vessels in a bloody wound must be avoided because of the potential for irreversible neurovascular damage. Similarly a tourniquet to control bleeding should be used with extreme caution because of the risk of ischemic injury to tissues distal to the tourniquet.

Certain hand injuries require emergent consultation with a hand specialist (orthopaedic surgeon or plastic surgeon). These conditions include major lacerations with arterial hemorrhage, complete or partial amputations of the digits, high-pressure injection injuries, thermal injuries, and compartment syndrome. These injuries must be evaluated and treated urgently to optimize recovery of function.

The decision to replant an amputated digit is a complex one that must be made by the treating surgeon after consideration of multiple factors, including the digit(s) involved, the level of amputation, the patient's age and functional demands, and the condition of the amputated part. The amputated part should be preserved, as previously described, pending this decision.

Replantation is not indicated for amputations through the distal phalanx (fingertip amputations). These relatively common injuries are managed effectively in the emergency department with debridement of the open wound, including bone as necessary, and loose closure of the soft tissues over the amputated tip. In general, good functional results can be anticipated following these injuries.

High-pressure injection injuries and thermal injuries initially may have a relatively benign appearance. It must be remembered, however, that these conditions left untreated can rapidly cause extensive tissue damage. Urgent operative debridement is necessary to avoid progressive tissue injury, which may result in amputation. Compartment syndrome of the hand requires emergent fasciotomy. Compartment syndromes are discussed in more detail in Chapter 32.

Orthopaedic or plastic surgery consultation is indicated for all fractures and dislocations of the hand. Urgent reduction is necessary for all dislocations. Most interphalangeal and metacarpophalangeal joint dislocations can be reduced with local anesthesia and closed techniques. Dislocations of the carpometacarpal joints are much less common; however, when present they usually require operative reduction and stabilization.

Most isolated metacarpal and phalangeal fractures are treated nonoperatively with a brief period of immobilization followed by early range of motion exercises (Fig. 25–1). Certain isolated metacarpal fractures (e.g., Bennett's fracture at base of thumb metacarpal), multiple metacarpal fractures, and intraarticular phalangeal fractures often are treated with operative reduction and fixation.

Consultation with a hand specialist also is indicated for open fracture or intraarticular open injury. Such injuries usually are treated with operative debridement or joint exploration and irrigation because of the increased risk of deep infection. One exception to this is the common open tuft fracture of the distal aspect of the distal phalanx. This injury can be managed effectively in the emergency department with debridement, irrigation, and loose closure of the skin laceration. Other open fracture wounds should be covered with a sterile povidone-iodine (Betadine)-soaked gauze dressing pending definitive treatment.

Fortunately most hand injuries can be managed effectively in the emergency department or outpatient setting. This includes the

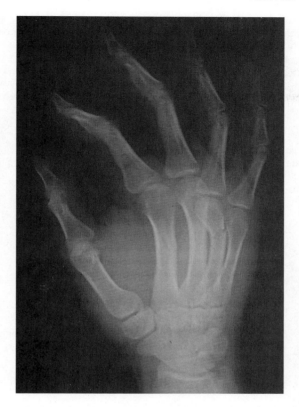

Figure 25–1 □ AP radiograph of the hand demonstrating a fracture of the ring finger metacarpal. This fracture is managed effectively nonoperatively.

common jammed finger injury, which represents a sprain to the supporting ligaments of the interphalangeal joints of the digits. These injuries are managed effectively with brief immobilization of the digit with an aluminum splint, followed by early motion exercises once the acute swelling and pain have subsided.

For lacerations with potential neurovascular or tendon damage and for injuries to the nailbed, evaluation and management in the emergency department is appropriate. Orthopaedic or plastic surgery consultation usually is necessary however. Lacerations should be irrigated, debrided of devitalized tissue, and loosely closed. As with all lacerations, the patient's tetanus status should be confirmed. The patient is also commonly discharged with a short course of an oral antibiotic (e.g., cephalexin 500 mg qid for 5 days). Nailbed injuries are treated with repair of the matrix and eponychium to preserve function and aesthetic appearance.

In the absence of fracture, dislocation, or laceration, hand injuries are treated symptomatically. Suspected sprains with swelling and localized joint tenderness can be treated with a brief period of immobilization (aluminum splint). Early motion should be encouraged, and NSAIDs used for alleviation of discomfort.

26

INABILITY TO MOVE THE FINGERS

C. Michael LeCroy

Inability to move one or more digits is a relatively common complaint following trauma to the upper extremity. Any of a wide variety of causes may be responsible, representing injury at different levels of the extremity or even the cervical spine. The most important initial determination to be made by the examiner is whether the patient *cannot* or *will not* move the finger(s). Not infrequently, patients with injury to the upper extremity will not move their fingers because of apprehension or pain. A thorough physical examination, combined with a detailed neurologic assessment of the extremity, is necessary to establish the correct diagnosis.

■ PHONE CALL

Questions

1. **How did the injury occur?**
    An understanding of the mechanism of injury is critical in the evaluation of musculoskeletal trauma. This is the first step in the formulation of a differential diagnosis.
2. **Is there obvious deformity?**
    Gross deformity of the upper extremity usually indicates fracture or dislocation, injuries that may be responsible for the disturbance in upper extremity motor function.
3. **Does the patient complain of pain in the affected upper extremity or neck?**
    Complaints of localized pain can be helpful in determining the musculoskeletal injury responsible for the inability to move the fingers.
4. **Is there an associated skin wound or laceration?**
    An open upper extremity wound should alert the physician to the potential for direct peripheral nerve injury or tendon laceration. In addition, such wounds may indicate an open fracture.
5. **Is the patient unable to move one, several, or all of the fingers?**
    This information can help determine the type of musculoskeletal injury or level of neurologic deficit responsible for the inability to move one or more fingers. For example, complete paralysis of the hand usually indicates a high neurologic lesion, whereas inability to move an isolated finger usually indicates a nonneurologic injury (e.g., tendon laceration).

6. Can the patient move the wrist? the elbow?

Spontaneous or voluntary movements of the affected upper extremity proximal to the fingers also will enable a rough assessment of the level of potential neurologic deficit.

7. Does the patient have sensation in the affected fingers?

Numbness in the hand and fingers can assist in determining the level of neurologic injury.

8. Are there any associated injuries (to other organ systems)?

As with all trauma to the musculoskeletal system, associated injuries to other body systems must be excluded. This is particularly important in cases of high-energy trauma, in which the incidence of associated injuries is high.

9. Is the patient hemodynamically stable?

Hemodynamic stability is the first priority of management in all trauma victims. If the patient is not hemodynamically stable, attention should be turned to the ABCs (airway, breathing, circulation) before the musculoskeletal injury is evaluated.

Orders

1. If obvious swelling or deformity is noted in the upper extremity, ask the RN to immobilize the area of injury by applying a shoulder immobilizer or elevating the forearm and hand on a pillow.
2. If there is a skin laceration in the upper extremity, ask the RN to apply a sterile compressive dressing.
3. If the patient has sustained a high-energy mechanism of injury, such as a motor vehicle accident, ask the RN to obtain immediate consultation with a general trauma specialist (emergency medicine physician or general surgeon).

Inform RN

"I will arrive at the bedside within 30 minutes."

Inability to move the fingers, whether due to pain and apprehension or to an actual anatomic lesion, indicates a significant injury to the musculoskeletal system. Although such injuries usually are not life or limb threatening, all patients with this complaint should be evaluated as soon as possible. If blood loss is ongoing or compartment syndrome of the forearm or hand is suspected, immediate evaluation is indicated. In general, to optimize outcome and minimize patient discomfort, all injuries to the upper extremity should be evaluated on an urgent basis.

■ ELEVATOR THOUGHTS

- Pain and apprehension
  - Patients with fractures or dislocations of the upper extremity may appear to be unable to move their fingers despite intact neurologic and tendon function.

- Dislocations (neurologic injury)
  - Shoulder dislocation (brachial plexus injury)
  - Elbow dislocation (median or ulnar nerve injury)
- Long bone fractures of upper extremity (neurologic injury)
  - Proximal humerus fracture (brachial plexus injury)
  - Humeral shaft fracture (radial nerve injury)
  - Distal humerus fracture (median or ulnar nerve injury)
  - Radial or ulnar fractures (median or ulnar nerve injury)
- High neurologic injuries
  - Lower cervical spine injury (involvement of C7, C8, T1 nerve roots)
  - Brachial plexus injury
- Isolated peripheral nerve injuries
  - Median nerve injury
  - Ulnar nerve injury
  - Radial nerve injury
- Tendon lacerations
  - Flexor tendon injury
  - Extensor tendon injury
- Other
  - Compartment syndrome of forearm
  - Compartment syndrome of hand

■ BEDSIDE

Vital Signs

A complete set of vital signs is indicated in all trauma patients. It must be remembered that inability to move the fingers heralds significant musculoskeletal injury, which can be expected to elevate the blood pressure and pulse rate. The blood pressure should not be checked in the injured upper extremity.

Selective History

How exactly did the injury occur?

Once the preliminary assessment is completed and hemodynamic stability has been assured, attention should be turned to a thorough investigation of the mechanism of injury. An understanding of the mechanism of injury can help to quickly narrow the differential diagnosis in the patient who is unable to move his or her fingers. For example, a patient with one or more lacerations to the extremity likely has sustained injury to peripheral nerves or tendons. On the other hand, a victim of a high-speed motor vehicle crash without associated lacerations may have sustained a lower cervical spine injury or a traction injury to the brachial plexus. Any high-energy trauma to the upper extremity may cause a fracture or dislocation that can be associated with secondary peripheral nerve injury. A patient who has sustained a significant crushing injury to the forearm or hand with subsequent inability to move the fingers should be considered at high risk for a compartment syndrome.

Can the patient localize any associated pain?

After the mechanism of injury has been determined, the patient should be asked to localize any concomitant symptoms of pain in the neck, shoulder, or upper extremity. Pain localized to the neck or shoulder points toward a high neurologic injury as the source of the paresis in the hand. Symptoms localized to the long bones or joints may implicate fracture or dislocation as the causative factor.

What are the patient-specific factors?

As with all injuries to the upper extremity, knowledge of factors specific to each individual patient is vital. These factors include the age of the patient, the handedness (i.e., right vs. left) of the patient, and any preexisting medical illnesses or conditions. In most cases this information will not establish the diagnosis; however, it is quite useful in formulating a plan of treatment and prognosis once the diagnosis has been established. Occasionally this simple questioning will reveal that the patient has a preexisting medical condition or injury, such as an old flexor tendon laceration, that explains the paresis in the hand.

Selective Physical Examination

Inspection

All clothing and jewelry should be removed to allow complete visual inspection of the neck, shoulder, and entire upper extremity. The location of any lacerations should be noted. Areas of swelling or deformity should be identified and comparison made to the uninjured upper extremity. The position or attitude of the involved digits should be noted: are the digits held in a position of flexion or extension? This may assist in establishing a diagnosis of flexor tendon injury (digit held in extension) or extensor tendon injury (digit held in flexion).

Palpation

The posterior neck, shoulder, and entire upper extremity should be palpated systematically, beginning centrally at the neck and proceeding peripherally to the digits of the injured extremity. Movement of fractured bone ends usually can be appreciated in the upper extremity with gentle palpation. All areas of tenderness should be noted and an attempt made to correlate these areas with the underlying anatomic structures. Diffuse and marked swelling of the entire forearm or hand following a crushing injury may indicate a developing compartment syndrome.

Movements

Assessment of movement in the injured extremity is, along with the neurologic examination, the most important step in the evaluation of the patient with inability to move the fingers. It is critical to determine whether the patient is unable to move the digit(s) because of an anatomic lesion or is unwilling to do so because of pain and apprehension. The patient should be encouraged to move the involved digit(s), even if only slightly. If necessary, intravenous analgesic medication may be administered to assist with the examination. All digits should be evaluated for both active flexion and extension. If a flexor tendon injury is suspected, active flexion of both the proximal (flexor digitorum superficialis) and distal (flexor digitorum profundus) interphalangeal joints must be evaluated separately to determine whether one or both flexor tendons are transected.

Every attempt should be made to determine whether one or several digits are involved in the paresis, as weakness isolated to a single digit narrows the differential diagnosis considerably. Given the patterns of innervation in the upper extremity, the physician should remember that it is not possible for a neurologic injury to cause paresis in a single finger (one possible exception: median nerve injury at the wrist, which can cause isolated thumb weakness). Thus, weakness isolated to a single digit generally points to a nonneurologic injury.

Gentle range of motion should be evaluated in all joints of the involved digit(s) as well as the elbow and shoulder to rule out dislocation. If compartment syndrome of the forearm or hand is suspected as the source of the weakness in the hand, the digits should be evaluated for pain with passive stretch. As described in Chapter 32, this is the most sensitive test for compartment syndrome.

Neurologic Examination

A thorough neurologic examination is the crux of the evaluation of the patient with inability to move the fingers. A complete understanding of the anatomy and patterns of innervation in the upper extremity is essential. It must be remembered that movement of the fingers is under the control of the C7, C8, and T1 nerve roots centrally (Fig. 26–1) and the median, ulnar, and radial nerves peripherally. A patient with suspected lower cervical spine or brachial plexus injury should be evaluated with respect to nerve root function in the upper extremity (high neurologic lesion). The following quick screening tests are helpful:

C7 Nerve Root
Motor: finger extension (metacarpophalangeal joint)
Sensory: long finger

C8 Nerve Root
Motor: finger flexion
Sensory: ring and small fingers

T1 Nerve Root

Motor: finger abduction and adduction
Sensory: medial aspect of arm proximal to elbow

A patient with a suspected peripheral nerve injury, either isolated or in association with a fracture or dislocation, should be examined specifically for the integrity of peripheral nerve function. To eliminate confusion caused by nonneurologic injuries to individual digits, each peripheral nerve function should be assessed in more than one digit. For example, a patient with absent PIP joint flexion in the long finger but intact thumb IP joint flexion cannot have a median nerve injury at the elbow level. The following screening tests are useful:

Median Nerve

Motor: thumb IP joint flexion, PIP joint flexion index, long, ring, and small fingers
Sensory: radial three and one-half digits

Ulnar Nerve

Motor: finger abduction and adduction, thumb adduction
Sensory: ulnar one and one-half digits

Radial Nerve

Motor: finger extension (MCP joints), thumb IP joint extension
Sensory: dorsal thumb web space

If the neurologic status of the extremity is found to be intact, tendon injury(ies) can be implicated as the source of the inability to move the finger(s).

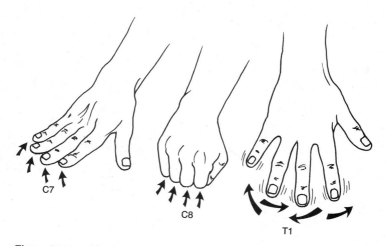

Figure 26–1 □ Movement of the fingers is under the control of the C7, C8, and T1 nerve roots centrally. (From Browner BD, Jupiter JB, Levine AM, Trafton PG: Skeletal Trauma. Philadelphia, WB Saunders, p 594.)

■ FURTHER ORDERS

No standard radiographs are indicated in the evaluation of the patient with inability to move the fingers. If fracture or dislocation is suspected on the basis of the history and physical examination, routine screening radiographs of the suspected injury area should be obtained.

■ MANAGEMENT

The immediate management of the patient with an inability to move the fingers should be directed at controlling ongoing bleeding from skin lacerations and immobilizing fractures and dislocations. Techniques for hemorrhage control and upper extremity immobilization, as outlined in preceding chapters, should be used.

A determination must be made as to whether the patient is physically unable or simply unwilling to move the finger or fingers in question. Patients with pain and apprehension but no anatomic explanation for their paresis should be managed with analgesic medications and primary attention to the injury causing the significant pain.

If the patient is felt to have a true inability to move one or more fingers, urgent orthopaedic consultation is indicated. The anatomic lesion should be identified and appropriate treatment initiated. Cervical spine injuries, shoulder or elbow dislocations, and upper extremity fractures should be managed as described in earlier chapters. In the presence of these injuries the paresis in the hand can be assumed to be due to a neurologic injury associated with the fracture or dislocation. In most cases this injury represents a neurapraxia rather than a complete nerve laceration, and the prognosis for recovery of function is good with expectant treatment.

If the patient has an isolated peripheral nerve injury due to a complex laceration, the prognosis for recovery of function is less certain. Orthopaedic consultation is indicated in all cases. Operative wound exploration with attempted peripheral nerve repair generally is indicated.

Tendon lacerations in the upper extremity account for a significant number of cases of finger weakness. The possibility of a tendon laceration should be anticipated with any laceration to the forearm or particularly to the hand. Consultation with a hand specialist (orthopaedic or plastic surgeon) should be obtained with all tendon lacerations. Extensor tendon lacerations are less complex and generally can be treated in the emergency department with simple repair. On the other hand, flexor tendon injuries are notoriously complex and require operative reconstruction to optimize outcome. Flexor tendon repairs generally are performed on a semielective basis.

The management of compartment syndromes of the forearm and hand involves emergent fasciotomy. Compartment syndromes are discussed in more detail in Chapter 32.

27

BACK PAIN

C. Michael LeCroy

Back pain is the most commonly encountered musculoskeletal complaint in office practice. In many, if not most, cases, pain in the back is not related to significant injury. Back injury does occur, however, and has a variety of causes. Motor vehicle accidents continue to be the primary source of most such injuries, with falls and recreational accidents frequently being implicated as well. Injuries to the back range in severity from the common muscle strain to complex fracture-dislocations of the thoracic or lumbar spine. Fractures and dislocations of the thoracolumbar spine frequently are associated with other injuries to the musculoskeletal system and other organ systems.

Most back injuries are not associated with any neurologic deficit. Devastating neurologic injury, however, can follow dislocations or fractures of the spinal column. For this reason, in cases of possible thoracolumbar spinal trauma the back must be adequately immobilized until fracture, dislocation, or ligament injury has been ruled out radiographically. All complaints of back pain following high-energy trauma should be taken seriously, and urgent evaluation is indicated in all cases. Once significant bone or ligament injury has been ruled out, early symptomatic treatment and patient education are necessary to help prevent the dreaded late complication of back injury—chronic low back pain.

■ PHONE CALL

Questions

1. **How was the back injured?**

    An understanding of the mechanism of injury is critical in the evaluation of musculoskeletal trauma. This is the initial step in the formulation of a differential diagnosis.

2. **Can the patient localize the pain?**

    The ability of the patient to localize the pain to a specific region can be very helpful in establishing a diagnosis. Not uncommonly, however, patients with back trauma will present with diffuse pain.

3. **Can the patient move all four extremities?**

    Spontaneous or voluntary movements of the extremities can provide a quick assessment of whether there is concomitant neurologic injury. A complete neurologic assessment must be performed subsequently during physical examination of the patient.

4. **Does the patient complain of numbness or tingling in the legs or feet?**

Radicular-like symptoms of radiating pain and intermittent tingling can be signs of nerve root involvement.

5. **Has the thoracolumbar spine been immobilized?**

In patients complaining of posttraumatic back pain, particularly following high-energy trauma, the thoracolumbar spine should be immobilized pending clinical and radiographic evaluation.

6. **Was the patient ambulatory after the injury occurred?**

A history of ambulation following injury makes significant thoracolumbar fracture or dislocation unlikely.

7. **Does the patient have any associated injuries?**

As with all trauma to the musculoskeletal system, associated injuries to the axial skeleton as well as to other body systems must be excluded. This is particularly true for high-energy spinal trauma, in which the incidence of associated injuries is high.

8. **Is the patient hemodynamically stable?**

Hemodynamic stability is the first priority of management in all trauma victims. If the patient is not hemodynamically stable, attention should be turned to the ABCs (airway, breathing, circulation) before the musculoskeletal injury is evaluated.

Orders

1. If the back has not been immobilized previously, take immediate steps to ensure that the thoracolumbar spine is adequately protected in all patients who have sustained documented back injury. Most commonly, this entails placing the patient supine on a rigid spine board. When placing or removing a spine board, assistance is necessary and care must be taken to logroll the patient so that the entire spine and torso move as a single unit. A rigid cervical collar should be applied to protect the cervical spine in all patients requiring protective immobilization of the thoracolumbar spine.

2. If the patient has sustained a high-energy mechanism of injury, such as a motor vehicle accident, ask the RN to obtain immediate consultation with a trauma specialist (emergency medicine physician or general surgeon).

Inform RN

"I will arrive at the bedside or emergency department immediately."

All back injuries should be evaluated immediately because of the potential for neurologic sequelae and the high incidence of associated injuries.

■ ELEVATOR THOUGHTS

Strains (Paraspinal Muscle Injuries)
- Thoracic strain
- Low back (lumbar) strain

Sprains
- Thoracolumbar spine ligament injury

Dislocations and Fractures
- Minor injuries
  - Articular process fracture
  - Transverse process fracture
  - Spinous process fracture
  - Pars interarticularis fracture
  - Vertebral body compression fracture
- Major injuries
  - Vertebral body burst fracture
  - Chance fracture (flexion-distraction injury)
  - Fracture-dislocation

Other
- Traumatic intervertebral disk herniation

■ BEDSIDE

Quick Look Test

Does the patient look well (comfortable), sick (uncomfortable or distressed), or critical (about to die)?

Patients who have sustained an injury to the back may have associated and potentially life-threatening injuries. Patients with back pain following trauma almost always are distressed and in varying degrees of acute pain. Brief observation of the supine patient can be helpful in detecting spontaneous movement of the lower extremities, which is a rough indication the patient does not have complete paralysis.

Vital Signs

Complete vital signs are essential in evaluating the patient with back injury to assure hemodynamic stability. In addition, in cases of high-energy trauma, monitoring of vital signs should be ongoing during the initial evaluation. Because of the potential for concomitant chest trauma, it is helpful to monitor oxygenation with a pulse oximeter. As in the evaluation of all injured patients, the basic principle of the ABCs is critical:

A: maintain airway
B: ensure adequate breathing or respirations
C: ensure adequate circulation

Selective History

How exactly was the back injured?

Once the preliminary assessment is completed and hemodynamic stability has been assured, a more detailed assessment of the mechanism of injury should be undertaken. An understanding of what caused the injury often will lead to an anatomic diagnosis. For example, in the case of a motor vehicle accident, answers to the following questions can be helpful: How did the accident occur (e.g., head-on collision or rollover)? Was the patient the driver or a passenger? Front seat or back seat? Was the patient restrained? Was the patient ejected from the vehicle? Patients sustaining frontal impact are more likely to experience fracture-dislocations of the thoracolumbar spine, whereas those involved in a rollover mechanism are more likely to have compression or burst fractures of the vertebral bodies. Likewise, the issue of seat belt restraint is critical, as restrained patients are more likely to experience flexion-distraction (Chance) injuries to the thoracolumbar spine.

What was the condition of the patient immediately following the injury?

Another useful piece of information is the status of the patient immediately following the accident or injury. Was the patient conscious throughout? Was the patient moving spontaneously at the scene? Was the patient ambulatory at the scene? If the patient is unable to provide this information, it often can be obtained from witnesses to the accident or from emergency medical personnel. These details allow a more accurate assessment of the severity of the injury to the thoracolumbar spine. For example, patients ambulatory at the scene generally do not have a significant fracture or dislocation.

What is the precise location of the pain?

The patient should be asked to localize the pain. This is often difficult, as back injury may be associated with diffuse pain. Any ability of the patient to localize the pain, however, can assist greatly in the subsequent physical and radiographic examinations. The patient also should be questioned regarding numbness, burning, or tingling in the lower extremities—symptoms that suggest nerve root irritation.

Is there a history of disease or injury in the back?

Finally, in the evaluation of injury to the back, it is especially important to elicit any history of spinal trauma or degenerative disease. This will allow acute injury to be distinguished from preexisting disease. Factors specific to the individual patient are equally critical in determining the course of treatment and prognosis and should be ascertained during this portion of the evaluation. These include the patient's occupation and functional demands, as well as the presence of any comorbid factors and preexisting medical conditions.

Selective Physical Examination

Inspection

Much useful information often can be gained by simply observing the patient lying supine on the stretcher or spine board. The degree of discomfort the patient is experiencing can be assessed. Most patients with a major fracture or dislocation of the thoracolumbar spine will complain of severe pain at the site of injury. This must be distinguished from the general discomfort almost all patients experience when lying on a rigid spine board. The patient also should be observed for movement. Spontaneous movement of the lower extremities almost always will be noted in patients without neurologic injury, regardless of associated injuries. Finally, the patient also should be inspected quickly from head to toe for deformity or abnormality of the head, trunk, and extremities.

Palpation

Many victims of trauma, particularly those involved in high-energy motor vehicle accidents, arrive in the emergency department lying supine on a rigid spine board. A significant number of these patients will report no back pain on initial questioning. In these patients a gentle logroll maneuver will allow visual inspection and palpation of the posterior elements of the thoracolumbar spine. The posterior spine should be palpated carefully from the upper thoracic region to the lumbosacral junction, searching for localized tenderness, crepitation, or stepoff between adjacent vertebral segments. If the patient has no complaint of back pain and no tenderness to palpation, the spine board can be removed safely.

If the patient does complain of back pain, palpation should be performed also. Adequate assistance is necessary to perform a careful, controlled logroll maneuver. The head and neck must be moved in unison with the torso. The back is palpated quickly but systematically, searching for points of localized tenderness, stepoff between adjacent vertebral segments, and paraspinal muscle tenderness (distinguished from midline tenderness). In patients with back pain or tenderness to palpation the wisest course is to leave the spine board in place pending review of radiographs.

Because of the high incidence of associated injuries in patients with thoracolumbar spine trauma, it is imperative that all patients with suspected back injury undergo a systematic examination with palpation from head to toe during the initial evaluation to rule out such associated injuries.

Neurologic Examination

All patients sustaining a back injury must have a complete neurologic examination, including evaluation of motor, sensory, and reflex function. It usually is easy for the examiner to identify major neurologic injury such as paraplegia; however, it is often difficult to identify accurately more subtle neurologic deficits. In cases of neurologic injury, it is critical to locate precisely the level of the neurologic deficit. Thus a systematic examination of the trunk and both lower extremities is necessary to assess integrity of thoracic, lumbar, and sacral nerve root function. By convention the level of neurologic injury is defined as the lowest level of intact nerve root function.

If there is neurologic injury, the trunk (chest and abdominal regions) should be examined for sensation. If the patient is moving the lower extremities, indicating intact thoracolumbar neurologic function, this sensory examination of the trunk usually is not necessary. For quick reference the following thoracic sensory levels are useful to remember:

T4: nipples

T10: umbilicus

T12: inguinal ligament

The lower extremities must be systematically examined for motor, sensory, and reflex function. Motor function should be graded using the standard scheme (Table 21–1). The following list describes the major motor, sensory, and reflex functions of the nerve roots in the lower extremities:

L1, L2, L3 *motor:* hip flexion

sensory: anterior thigh just below inguinal ligament (**L1**)

anterior aspect midthigh (**L2**)

anterior thigh just above patella (**L3**)

reflex: none

L4 *motor:* dorsiflexion of ankle

sensory: medial aspect of lower leg

reflex: patellar tendon

L5 *motor:* dorsiflexion of great toe

sensory: lateral aspect of lower leg, dorsum of foot

reflex: posterior tibial tendon

S1 *motor:* ankle eversion and plantar flexion

sensory: sole of foot, lateral malleolus of ankle

reflex: Achilles tendon

Patients with documented neurologic deficit following back injury also should be evaluated for *spinal shock.* The exact level of neurologic injury cannot be specified so long as the patient remains in spinal shock, which may last for 24 to 72 hours following thoracolumbar spinal trauma. Spinal shock may be determined with the bulbocavernosus reflex (anal sphincter contraction in response to squeezing the glans penis or pulling on the Foley catheter). The return of the bulbocavernosus reflex signifies the end of spinal shock, and further neurologic improvement in most cases will be minimal.

■ FURTHER ORDERS

All patients who have sustained a back injury must undergo radiographic evaluation of the thoracolumbar spine. A standard thoracolumbar spine trauma series includes AP and lateral images of the thoracic and lumbosacral spine. It is important to remember that the entire thoracolumbar spine cannot be adequately visualized on a single radiograph in either the coronal or sagittal plane. To radiographically "clear" the spine, all vertebral segments from the cervicothoracic to the lumbosacral junctions must be visualized. If the level of injury is suspected from the physical examination findings, it is particularly helpful to obtain a lateral radiograph centered at this level. Occasionally oblique radiographs of the lumbosacral spine also are indicated in the evaluation of spinal trauma to rule out fractures of the articular processes or pars interarticularis.

■ MANAGEMENT

All complaints of back pain following injury must be taken seriously. If the patient has sustained a high-energy injury, such as a motor vehicle crash or fall from a height, the thoracolumbar spine should be protected on a rigid spine board during the initial examination and radiographic evaluation. If the patient must be turned, a logroll maneuver should prevent torsional force to the spinal column. The purpose of these procedures and precautions is to protect against causing or worsening a neurologic injury in an unstable thoracolumbar spine. Every attempt should be made to evaluate the back injury expeditiously and remove the spine board as soon as it is safe to do so to prevent pressure necrosis and to improve patient comfort. As a general rule the safest course of action is to have the thoracolumbar spine "cleared" by a trauma specialist or spine specialist. This must be an individual experienced in the interpretation of thoracolumbar spine films and the treatment of potential injuries to the bony and ligamentous structures of the back.

Orthopaedic or neurosurgical consultation should be requested immediately for all patients with abnormal neurologic examination findings or abnormalities on radiographs. In most cases the consultant will recommend additional radiographic studies to delineate the injury pattern more clearly. This most commonly involves a CT scan but also may include an MRI scan or myelography. These additional studies will enable the treating spine specialist to characterize the bone and ligament injury and to determine the stability of the spinal column injury.

Minor fractures of the thoracolumbar spine generally can be managed nonoperatively with symptomatic treatment. These injuries, in the absence of associated fracture or ligament injury, are stable. Patients should be treated with appropriate analgesic medication and allowed to be out of bed as soon as comfortable. Bracing for these isolated minor fractures rarely is indicated.

Compression fractures of the thoracolumbar spine involve the anterior column of the spinal segment only and are inherently stable. Symptomatic treatment is indicated with analgesic medication, early mobilization, and close follow-up. Bracing for these injuries is not necessary under most circumstances. An upright lateral radiograph should be obtained as soon as the patient is ambulatory to confirm stability of the spinal column.

Vertebral body burst fractures (Fig. 27–1) by definition involve the anterior and middle columns of the spinal segment and may

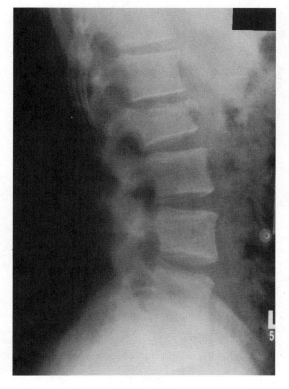

Figure 27–1 □ Lateral lumbosacral spine radiograph illustrating an L2 burst fracture.

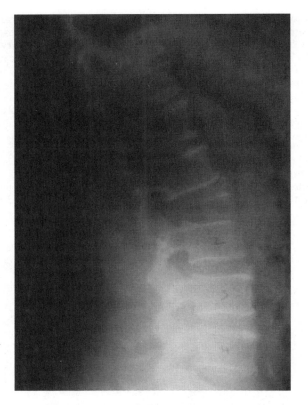

Figure 27–2 □ Lateral lumbosacral spine radiograph illustrating a fracture-dislocation at the L1–2 level.

include retropulsion of bone into the spinal canal. These injuries have the potential for significant instability and neurologic injury. Many burst fractures may be managed nonoperatively in a rigid thoracolumbosacral orthosis (TLSO), using established radiographic criteria for anterior vertebral body height loss, degree of canal compromise, and amount of relative kyphosis at the involved level. The decision for nonoperative vs. operative treatment of burst fractures is complex and should be made by a spine specialist on a case-by-case basis with consideration given to the spine injury as well as to associated injuries and preexisting illnesses.

Chance fractures of the thoracolumbar spine occur with flexion-distraction forces. The most common mechanism is seatbelt (lap-belt) injury. These injuries involve the anterior, middle, and posterior columns of the spine and are unstable. Pure bony Chance fractures may be managed nonoperatively in a rigid hyperextension orthosis. Ligamentous and mixed bony-ligamentous Chance fractures, on the other hand, usually are managed best with operative stabilization.

Fracture-dislocations of the thoracolumbar spine involve all three columns and are inherently unstable (Fig. 27–2). These injuries characteristically present with neurologic deficit—usually paraplegia below the level of injury. Most fracture-dislocations are managed with operative stabilization.

Traumatic disk herniation in the thoracic and lumbar spine is uncommon. It should be suspected in patients with pain, paresthesias, and neurologic deficit following back injury but with negative radiographs. The diagnosis can be made using either an MRI scan or myelography. The treatment usually is surgical decompression with excision of the herniated disk.

Fortunately most cases of back pain following trauma do not involve significant bone or ligament injury and are not associated with neurologic deficit. These strains and sprains will present with negative radiographs and normal neurologic examinations. The treatment of these injuries is symptomatic. Pharmacologic treatment should consist of NSAIDs and possibly a brief course of a mild antispasmodic agent. As with nontraumatic back pain, narcotic analgesics should be avoided because of the potential for abuse and addiction. Application of heat to the paraspinal muscles is often helpful, and a structured physical therapy program for stretching and muscle conditioning should be initiated as soon as possible. Relative rest for the spine also is indicated, with the patient being instructed to avoid heavy lifting and vigorous physical activity. Strict bed rest, however, should be avoided because of the potential for muscle weakness and prolonged recovery time.

Finally, an important, but often overlooked, component of the treatment of back strains and sprains is patient education. Patients should be counseled and reassured regarding the good prognosis and the absence of potential for paralysis. All the above measures are important and when instituted in timely fashion may prevent the progression of acute back strain to chronic low back pain.

28

PELVIC PAIN

C. Michael LeCroy

Injury to the pelvic ring usually is caused by high-energy trauma, such as a motor vehicle accident or a fall from a height. It is rare for a patient to complain of true pelvic pain following low-energy trauma. The pelvic ring is a complex anatomic structure with numerous bony articulations, supporting ligaments, and muscle attachments. For this reason, pelvic pain may originate from a variety of injuries. As with trauma to the remainder of the axial skeleton (neck and back), there is a high incidence of associated injuries in patients sustaining pelvic trauma. Most pelvic ring injuries have a benign clinical course and are associated with good outcomes. Unstable pelvic ring disruptions, however, can be life threatening and can result in significant long-term disability.

■ PHONE CALL

Questions

1. **How was the pelvic ring injured?**
   An understanding of the mechanism of injury is critical in the evaluation of musculoskeletal trauma. This is the initial step in the formulation of a differential diagnosis.
2. **Is there gross deformity?**
   Obvious deformity of the pelvis or lower extremities usually indicates fracture or dislocation.
3. **Can the patient localize the pain, and if so, where?**
   The ability of the patient to localize the pain to a specific region of the pelvis can be helpful in establishing a diagnosis.
4. **Is there an associated skin wound or laceration?**
   An open wound should alert the physician to the potential for an open fracture, which requires urgent evaluation and treatment.
5. **Can the patient move the lower extremities?**
   Spontaneous or voluntary movements of the lower extremities distal to the site of injury can provide a rough assessment of whether there is concomitant neurologic injury. This must be evaluated subsequently by physical examination.
6. **Was the patient ambulatory after the injury occurred?**
   A history of ambulation following injury makes significant pelvic ring disruption highly unlikely.

7. **Is the patient complaining of numbness or tingling in the legs or feet?**

Complaints of numbness or paresthesias in one or both lower extremities following pelvic trauma can be a sign of neurologic injury.

8. **Does the patient have any associated injuries?**

As with all trauma to the musculoskeletal system, associated injuries to other body systems must be ruled out. This is particularly important in cases of high-energy pelvic trauma, in which the incidence of associated injuries is high.

9. **Is the patient hemodynamically stable?**

Hemodynamic stability is the first priority of management in all trauma victims. If the patient is not hemodynamically stable, attention should be turned to the ABCs (airway, breathing, circulation) before the musculoskeletal injury is evaluated.

Orders

1. All patients complaining of pelvic pain following trauma should be placed supine on a stretcher or hospital bed. The patient should not be allowed to ambulate. Because of the high incidence of concomitant injury to the axial skeleton, steps also should be taken to ensure adequate protection of the thoracolumbar spine with a rigid back board and of the cervical spine with a rigid cervical collar.
2. Ask the RN to obtain immediate consultation with a trauma specialist (emergency medicine physician or general surgeon). This is necessary because of the potential for significant injury to multiple organ systems in association with pelvic ring trauma, which usually results from a high-energy injury.

Inform RN

"I will arrive at the bedside immediately."

A complaint of pelvic pain following trauma requires that the patient be evaluated immediately because of the potential for life-threatening pelvic ring disruption as well as the high incidence of associated injuries.

■ ELEVATOR THOUGHTS

- Strains
    Abductor muscle strain
- Sprains
    Pubic symphyseal ligament injury
    Pubic symphysis disruption

- Dislocations
    Sacroiliac joint diastasis or disruption
- Fractures
    Coccygeal fracture
    Pubic rami fracture(s)
    Sacral fracture
    Iliac wing fracture
    Acetabular fracture

■ BEDSIDE

Quick Look Test

Does the patient look well (comfortable), sick (uncomfortable or distressed), or critical (about to die)?

A patient with an unstable pelvic ring disruption may develop life-threatening hemorrhage. In addition, other associated and potentially life-threatening injuries may be present. Almost all patients with pelvic pain following trauma will appear distressed and in varying degrees of acute pain. A quick observation of the supine patient can be helpful in detecting spontaneous movement of the lower extremities. This can assist the physician in determining the potential for concomitant neurologic injury.

Vital Signs

Complete vital signs are essential in evaluating the patient with pelvic injury to assure hemodynamic stability. In addition, it is recommended that monitoring of vital signs be ongoing during the initial evaluation of patients who have been the victims of high-energy trauma. Hypotension or significant tachycardia may herald hemorrhagic shock. As in the evaluation of all injuries, the ABCs are critical:

A: maintain airway
B: ensure adequate breathing or respirations
C: ensure adequate circulation

Selective History

How exactly was the pelvic ring injured?

Once the preliminary assessment is completed and hemodynamic stability has been assured, the exact mechanism of injury should be determined. The examiner should elicit as much detail regarding the injury as possible. Significant pelvic ring injury is usually the result of high-energy trauma such as motor vehicle crashes, falls from a height, or a direct blow to the pelvis. Each of these mechanisms is associated with a characteristic pelvic ring injury pattern, and thus an understanding of how the patient was injured often can lead to an anatomic diagnosis. For example, a patient involved in a head-on-collision motor vehicle accident may experience significant anteroposterior compression force to the pelvic ring with resulting disruption of the pubic symphysis and possibly the sacroiliac ligaments as well (open book pelvic fracture). Similarly a patient who falls from a height may experience vertical shear forces to the pelvic ring with resulting rami fractures and sacroiliac joint dislocation.

What was the condition of the patient following the injury?

It is also helpful to determine the condition of the patient immediately following the accident or injury. Was the patient conscious throughout? Was the patient moving spontaneously at the scene? Was the patient ambulatory at the scene? If the patient is unable to provide this information, it often can be obtained from witnesses to the accident or from emergency medical personnel. These details can assist the treating physician in assessing the potential for significant injury to the pelvic ring as well as other body systems. For example, a patient ambulatory at the scene of the accident is not likely to have a significant pelvic ring fracture or dislocation.

Can the patient localize the pain?

The patient should be asked to localize the pain. In many cases this will not be possible since pelvic ring injuries frequently present with diffuse pain. Not uncommonly, patients will indicate nonspecific pain in the region of the groin, which can be encountered in a wide variety of pelvic and hip injuries. On some occasions, however, the patient may be able to precisely localize the pain to, for example, the iliac wing. This information can be useful in the subsequent physical and radiographic examinations. The patient also should be questioned regarding any symptoms of numbness, tingling, or burning in the lower extremities, any of which could suggest nerve root irritation.

What are the patient-specific factors?

A final category of information that should be elicited during this portion of the evaluation includes factors specific to the patient. The age of the patient is important, as elderly patients are likely to sustain pelvic ring disruption at relatively lower energy mechanisms than are younger adults. Any prior pelvic injuries or disease should be identified so that acute trauma can be distinguished from a preexisting condition. The patient's occupation and functional demands should be determined, as well as any comorbid factors and chronic medical conditions. Although this information usually will not establish the diagnosis, it is useful in formulating a treatment plan and prognosis once the diagnosis has been made.

Selective Physical Examination

Inspection

The patient should be examined while disrobed, if possible, and lying supine on a stretcher or hospital bed. The degree of discomfort the patient is experiencing usually can be determined in a few seconds by simply observing the patient. Notation should be made of any deformity, swelling, ecchymosis, or skin laceration. In male patients the penis should be inspected for blood at the urethral meatus, which may indicate urogenital injury in association with a pelvic ring injury. The patient also should be observed for spontaneous movement of the lower extremities, which usually indicates intact neurologic status. Finally the patient should be inspected quickly for deformity or abnormality of the head, trunk, and extremities.

Palpation

The bony contours of the pelvic ring should be palpated in a systematic fashion. A thorough examination includes palpation of the pubic symphysis, anterior iliac spines, iliac crest, and sacrum. The pubic rami generally cannot be directly palpated because of overlying soft tissue structures; rami fractures, however, are characterized by tenderness in the region of the inguinal ligament. Any tenderness or crepitation along the bony pelvic ring can be indicative of a pelvic fracture and can help focus the subsequent radiographic examination.

In patients who have sustained suspected pelvic ring injury, the pelvis should be palpated for stability as part of the initial evaluation. This is accomplished using the bimanual compression test, which is performed by placing the examiner's thumbs over the anterior iliac spines and applying a gentle posteriorly directed force to both sides of the pelvic ring. Instability of the pelvic ring is characterized by pain and gross displacement of one hemipelvis relative to the other. As a general rule, if the pelvis is unstable either by the bimanual test or on the basis of the initial trauma pelvis radiograph, this maneuver should not be repeated because of the potential for disrupting fracture hematoma and causing hemorrhage.

Because of the high incidence of associated injuries in patients with pelvic ring trauma, it is imperative that all patients with suspected pelvic injury undergo a systematic examination with palpation from head to toe during the initial evaluation in an attempt to identify any associated injuries.

Movements

Pelvic pain, particularly that due to fracture of the acetabulum, can be difficult to differentiate from pain arising from injury to the hip joint (proximal femur). Nevertheless, patients with suspected pelvic injury should be examined with passive movement of the hip joints. Although significant pain or limited range of motion with this maneuver may not differentiate pelvic ring injury from hip trauma, it will serve to focus the radiographic examination. Patients with no pain and full range of motion can be assumed to have no fracture of the acetabulum or proximal femur.

Neurovascular Examination

All patients sustaining injury to the pelvic ring must have a complete neurologic examination to exclude injury to the lumbosacral nerve roots. The L4 and L5 nerve roots are particularly at risk because of their position just anterior to the sacroiliac articulation, and neurologic deficit may be encountered with fractures of the sacrum or sacroiliac joint disruptions. Evaluation of nerve root function in both lower extremities with motor, sensory, and reflex examinations is necessary to rule out nerve root or lumbosacral plexus injury. The following list describes the major motor, sensory, and reflex functions of the nerve roots in the lower extremities.

L1, L2, L3 *motor:* hip flexion
  sensory: anterior thigh just below inguinal ligament (**L1**)
    anterior aspect midthigh (**L2**)
    anterior thigh just above patella (**L3**)
  reflex: none
L4 *motor:* dorsiflexion of ankle
  sensory: medial aspect of lower leg
  reflex: patellar tendon
L5 *motor:* dorsiflexion of great toe
  sensory: lateral aspect of lower leg, dorsum of foot
  reflex: posterior tibial tendon
S1 *motor:* ankle eversion, plantar flexion of ankle
  sensory: lateral malleolus of ankle, sole of foot
  reflex: Achilles tendon

Motor function should be graded using the standard scheme (see Table 21–1).

Major intrapelvic arterial injury is relatively uncommon following pelvic ring trauma. The significant hemorrhage that may accompany these injuries usually is due to disruption of the large retroperitoneal pelvic venous plexuses. The adequacy of peripheral vascular perfusion can be assessed quickly through palpation of the dorsalis pedis or posterior tibial pulses at the dorsum of the foot or the medial malleolus, respectively. The physician should remember that the most common cause of absent or diminished pulses in the lower extremities following pelvic injury is hemorrhagic shock and not arterial injury.

■ FURTHER ORDERS

All patients who have sustained an injury to the pelvis must undergo radiographic evaluation of the pelvic ring. This is performed initially by obtaining an AP radiograph. All patients who have sustained a high-energy mechanism of trauma will require an AP pelvis radiograph, along with an AP chest film and a lateral cervical spine radiograph, as part of their initial trauma evaluation and resuscitation according to advanced trauma life support (ATLS) protocol.

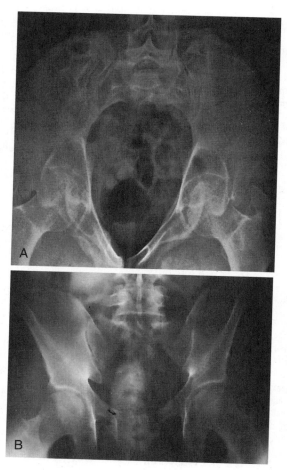

Figure 28–1 □ **A,** The inlet view of the pelvis, which allows assessment of anteroposterior displacement of the pelvic ring. **B,** The outlet view of the pelvis, which allows assessment of vertical displacement of the pelvic ring. (From Browner BD, Jupiter JB, Levine AM, Trafton PG: Skeletal Trauma. Philadelphia, WB Saunders, 1992, pp 870 and 871.)

The initial AP pelvis radiograph usually will allow the identification of significant bone or ligament disruptions of the pelvic ring. If pelvic ring injury is identified or suspected after review of the AP pelvis radiograph, and assuming the patient remains hemodynamically stable, it often is helpful to obtain inlet and outlet radiographs of the pelvic ring. The inlet view (Fig. 28–1A) allows assessment of anteroposterior displacement of the pelvic ring, whereas the outlet view (Fig. 28–1B) allows the identification of vertical migration of one hemipelvis relative to the other. These additional images are helpful in establishing the stability of the pelvic ring following injury. As an important aside, in the face of hemodynamic instability the urgent treatment of an unstable pelvic ring disruption should never be delayed for further radiographic evaluation.

■ MANAGEMENT

Pelvic pain following high-energy trauma should be evaluated on an urgent basis because of the potential for life-threatening hemorrhage as well as injury to other body systems. In addition to obtaining pertinent radiographs, the initial treating physician must take steps to ensure adequate protection of the pelvis and associated body systems. Gentle handling of the patient, with as little rolling or lifting as possible, is important for patient comfort as well as to avoid disruption of pelvic fracture hematoma. Patients should not be allowed to ambulate, or even sit up, until stability of the pelvic ring has been determined radiographically. Also, the potential for associated urogenital injury must be remembered. Patients with blood at the urethral meatus or vaginal vault should not undergo routine bladder catheterization pending urologic consultation and radiographic examination of the urogenital system.

Patients with abnormal pelvic radiographs or neurologic examination should have immediate orthopaedic consultation. In fractures and dislocations of the pelvic ring the first priority of the consultant is to establish the stability of the pelvis. In most cases the consultant will recommend additional radiographic studies to assist in this determination. Inlet and outlet plain radiographs of the pelvis may be obtained, as well as a pelvic CT scan with bone windows. The CT scan can be particularly helpful in the evaluation of fractures of the sacrum and the posterior sacroiliac ligaments (Fig. 28–2). If an acetabular fracture is identified on the initial AP pelvic radiograph, specialized oblique radiographs (Judet views) of the affected acetabulum are indicated. In addition, most acetabular fractures are evaluated further with thin cut CT scans (3 mm) to allow characterization of the acetabular fracture pattern.

Stable pelvic ring fractures are those that do not involve ligament disruption of the pubic symphysis anteriorly or the sacroiliac ligaments posteriorly. Examples of this group of injuries include most pubic rami fractures (the most common pelvic ring disruption encountered), iliac wing fractures, avulsion fractures of the iliac crest, and anterior sacral compression fractures. Most of these injuries can be treated symptomatically with analgesic medication and early weight bearing. Close orthopaedic follow-up is necessary, and it is recommended that orthopaedic consultation be obtained before ambulation is allowed in any patient with a pelvic ring fracture.

Unstable pelvic ring injuries involve disruption of the anterior or posterior ligamentous restraints of the pelvic ring. There may be associated fractures as well. These injuries are characterized as being rotationally unstable (e.g., open book pelvic fracture), vertically unstable, or both rotationally and vertically unstable. Unstable pelvic ring injuries will require, at a minimum, a period of protected weight bearing and close clinical and radiographic follow-up. Certain types of unstable pelvic ring disruptions are managed best with operative stabilization. The best example is that of the open book pelvic fracture associated with hemodynamic instability (Fig. 28–3), where application of a pelvic external fixator can be a life-saving maneuver. Various internal and external fixation techniques have been described for the treatment of the unstable pelvic ring, and the treatment of each injury is individualized based on the judgment and experience of the orthopaedic consultant as well as the specifics of the particular injury.

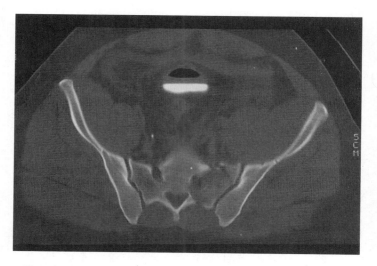

Figure 28–2 □ Pelvic CT scan illustrating fracture of the left sacrum.

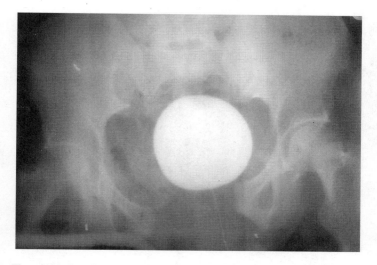

Figure 28–3 □ Anteroposterior compression injury of pelvic ring (open book pelvic fracture). Note wide diastasis of pubic symphysis and right sacroiliac joint.

Fractures of the acetabulum (Fig. 28–4) represent a unique and difficult challenge in orthopaedic trauma. Most orthopaedists believe that displaced fractures involving the major weight-bearing portion of the acetabular articular surface in active patients should be treated with operative reduction and stabilization. Surgery generally is performed on a semielective basis several days after the acute injury. Patients commonly are managed in skeletal traction via a tibial traction pin while awaiting operative intervention. Protected or non-weight-bearing status is required for the affected leg for 8 to 12 weeks following acetabular fracture, regardless of whether operative or nonoperative treatment is selected.

Abductor muscle strain injuries, pubic symphysis injuries without ligament disruption, and coccygeal fractures are treated symptomatically. The patient should be encouraged to resume weight bearing as soon as possible. NSAIDs are helpful in the management of acute pain and inflammation, and application of heat to the abductor muscles is often effective. A structured physical therapy program is rarely necessary with these injuries, although some patients may need assistance with ambulation in the acute period.

A final point regarding the management of pelvic ring disruptions involves the increased potential for deep venous thrombosis with these injuries. This increased risk is related both to venous disruption at the time of initial injury as well as the subsequent requirement for bedrest or relative immobilization. Fatal pulmonary

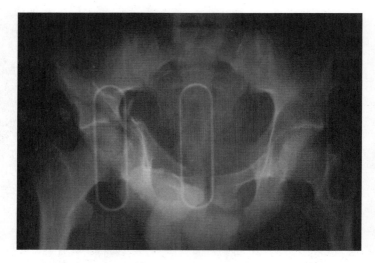

Figure 28–4 □ AP pelvis radiograph illustrating a complex fracture of the right acetabulum.

embolus has been reported following pelvic fracture; for this reason, prophylaxis is indicated for all patients with pelvic fractures requiring even a brief period of immobilization. The exact nature and duration of prophylaxis should be determined by the treating orthopaedic physician. Commonly used agents include sequential compression devices, warfarin, low-dose heparin, and low-molecular-weight heparins.

29

HIP AND THIGH PAIN

C. Michael LeCroy

In young adults, dislocation of the hip or fracture of the proximal femur or femoral shaft characteristically is the result of high-energy trauma such as a motor vehicle accident. On the other hand, in elderly patients, fracture of the proximal femur is not uncommon following low-energy mechanisms of injury such as simple falls. Although muscle strain injuries occur occasionally, many patients complaining of significant hip or thigh pain following trauma will be found to have a hip dislocation or, more commonly, a fracture of the proximal femur or femoral shaft. Often an accurate diagnosis can be made at the bedside through observation of the extremity and simple physical examination maneuvers. Because of significant advances in the treatment of fractures of the proximal femur and femoral shaft, these injuries carry a relatively good prognosis for early return to normal ambulation.

■ PHONE CALL

Questions

1. **How was the hip or thigh injured?**
   An understanding of the mechanism of injury is critical in the evaluation of musculoskeletal trauma. This is the initial step in the formulation of a differential diagnosis.
2. **Is there gross deformity?**
   Obvious deformity of the hip or thigh usually indicates fracture or dislocation or both.
3. **Can the patient localize the pain to a specific area?**
   The ability of the patient to localize the pain to a specific region of the hip or thigh can be very helpful in establishing a diagnosis.
4. **Is there an associated skin wound or laceration?**
   An open wound should alert the physician to the potential for an open fracture or intraarticular communication. These conditions require urgent evaluation and treatment.
5. **Can the patient move the affected lower extremity?**
   Spontaneous or voluntary movements of the extremity distal to the site of injury can provide a rough assessment of whether there is concomitant neurologic injury. This must be evaluated subsequently by physical examination.
6. **Can the patient ambulate on the injured lower extremity?**

A history of weight bearing on the injured leg makes hip dislocation or femoral fracture highly unlikely.

7. Are there any additional injuries?

As with all trauma to the musculoskeletal system, associated injuries to other body systems must be ruled out. This is particularly important in cases of high-energy trauma, in which the incidence of associated injuries is high.

8. Is the patient hemodynamically stable?

Hemodynamic stability is the first priority of management in all trauma victims. If the patient is not hemodynamically stable, attention should be turned to the ABCs (airway, breathing, circulation) before the musculoskeletal injury is evaluated.

Orders

1. Steps should be taken to ensure adequate immobilization of the involved extremity, particularly if evaluation of the patient is going to be delayed for any length of time. Immobilization helps prevent further damage to the soft tissues about the hip and thigh, and it is essential for patient comfort. Victims of high-energy trauma often will arrive in the emergency department with traction applied to the leg, usually via a Hare traction splint (Fig. 29–1A). In the absence of this temporary traction splint the hip and thigh can be effectively immobilized either by common Buck's traction (Fig. 29–1B) or by applying plaster or wooden splints to the medial and lateral aspects of the extremity.

2. If the patient has sustained a high-energy mechanism of injury, such as a motor vehicle accident, ask the RN to obtain immediate consultation with a trauma specialist (emergency medicine physician or general surgeon).

Inform RN

"I will arrive at the bedside within 30 minutes."

In the absence of other organ system injuries, injury to the hip or thigh usually is not life or limb threatening. Because of the potential for significant blood loss following fractures of the femoral shaft, however, these injuries should be evaluated on an urgent basis. Also, if an open fracture is suspected from the described injury mechanism and history, the patient should be evaluated emergently. In general, to minimize patient discomfort and optimize outcome, all injuries to the hip and thigh should be evaluated as soon as possible.

■ ELEVATOR THOUGHTS

Strains
- Adductor muscle strain
- Quadriceps muscle strain or contusion
- Hamstring muscle strain or avulsion

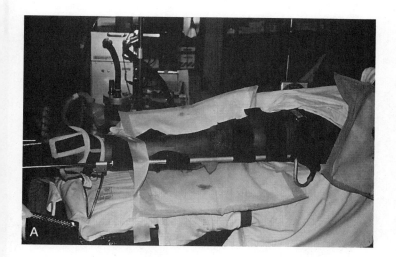

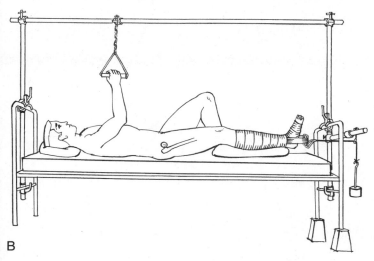

Figure 29–1 □ **A,** A Hare traction splint, which is used for temporary stabilization of femoral shaft fractures. **B,** Buck's skin traction, which is used for
immobilization of hip and thigh injuries. Five to ten pounds of traction typically is applied. (*A* from Browner BD, Jupiter JB, Levine AM, Trafton PG:
Skeletal Trauma. Philadelphia, WB Saunders, 1992, p 1543. *B* from
Schmeisser G Jr: A Clinical Manual of Orthopedic Traction Techniques.
Philadelphia, WB Saunders, 1963.)

Sprains
- None

Dislocations
- Hip dislocation

Fractures
- Proximal femur fractures
  Femoral head fracture
  Femoral neck fracture (Fig. 29–2A)

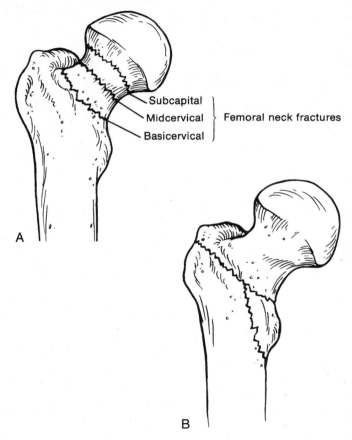

Figure 29–2 □ **A,** Types of femoral neck fractures. **B,** Location of intertrochanteric femur fracture. (From Wiesel SW, Delahay JN: Essentials of Orthopaedic Surgery, 2nd ed. Philadelphia, WB Saunders, 1997, pp 73 and 74.)

Greater trochanteric fracture
Intertrochanteric femur fracture (Fig. 29–2B)
Subtrochanteric femur fracture
- Femoral shaft fracture

Other
- Compartment syndrome of the thigh

■ BEDSIDE

Vital Signs

A complete set of vital signs must be obtained in any trauma victim. Patients with femoral shaft fracture may present with tachycardia and hypotension due to the significant hemorrhage associated with these injuries. In these patients the vital signs should be monitored continuously. In contrast, fractures of the proximal femur are not associated with blood loss and generally will not compromise the vital signs. In all musculoskeletal injuries, it should be anticipated that pain and anxiety will elevate the heart rate and blood pressure.

Selective History

How exactly was the hip or thigh injured?
Once the preliminary assessment is completed and hemodynamic stability has been assured, the examiner should attempt to elicit as much information regarding the mechanism of injury as possible. Often an understanding of how the injury occurred can lead to the correct diagnosis. For example, Was the patient involved in a frontal impact motor vehicle accident (common mechanism for hip dislocation or femoral shaft fracture)? Did the patient sustain a twisting injury to the hip or proximal thigh (femoral neck or subtrochanteric fracture)? Did the patient sustain a direct blow to the anterior thigh musculature (quadriceps contusion)? Was there a crushing injury to the thigh (risk for compartment syndrome)? This information also can alert the examiner to potential associated injuries to the musculoskeletal system as well as other organ systems.

What was the condition of the patient immediately following the injury?
It is also helpful to determine the condition of the patient immediately following the accident or injury. A particular point of interest is whether the patient was able to ambulate at the scene. This detail can assist the treating physician in assessing the potential for significant injury to the hip and femur, as a history of ambulation after injury is not consistent with a hip dislocation or femoral fracture.

Can the patient localize the pain?

The patient also should be asked to localize the pain. This may be helpful in differentiating a femoral shaft fracture from a fracture-dislocation of the proximal femur. Patients with hip fracture or dislocation characteristically will complain of pain in the groin area and not in the thigh itself. It should be noted, however, that groin pain is relatively nonspecific and can be encountered with a variety of hip and pelvic pathologic conditions. The patient should be questioned regarding numbness or tingling in the affected lower extremity—symptoms that suggest neurovascular injury.

What are the patient-specific factors?

An essential component of the history in the evaluation of trauma-induced hip and thigh pain is the preinjury condition of the patient. This is particularly critical in elderly patients in whom hip fracture is suspected. Every attempt should be made through questioning of the patient and the family to determine the premorbid functional status of the patient. Was the patient ambulatory or nonambulatory? If the patient is an ambulator, does she or he use any assistive device? Is the patient able to ambulate outside the home (community ambulator) or only inside the home (household ambulator). These details weigh heavily in the determination of treatment goals and prognosis for the elderly patient with a hip fracture. In elderly patients it is important to identify any history of prior hip injury or disease so that the acute trauma can be distinguished from a preexisting condition. In all patients, any comorbid factors or chronic medical conditions should be identified. Although this information usually will not establish the diagnosis, it is useful in formulating a treatment plan and prognosis once the diagnosis has been made.

Selective Physical Examination

Inspection

The patient should be disrobed, except for underwear, and lying supine on a stretcher or hospital bed. With injuries to the hip and thigh, much information can be gained through simple observation of the patient. The degree of discomfort the patient is experiencing should be noted. This may assist the physician in determining the potential for significant fracture or dislocation. In addition, careful attention should be paid to the position of the involved extremity. Dislocations of the hip and fractures of the proximal femur present with characteristic deformities, and the diagnosis occasionally can be made on this basis alone. In a posterior dislocation of the hip, flexion, adduction, and internal rotation of the hip and thigh will be noted. Conversely, in the much less common anterior dislocation of the hip, the extremity will be held in extension, abduction, and external rotation. Displaced fractures of the femoral neck present with shortening and external rotation of the extremity. Deformity of the thigh may be noted in fractures of the femoral shaft, with shortening of the thigh relative to the contralateral lower extremity.

Notation also should be made of any swelling, ecchymosis, or skin laceration. The communication of any wounds or lacerations with underlying fracture must be ruled out. Finally the patient is observed for spontaneous movements of the lower extremity, which usually indicate intact neurologic status.

Palpation

The hip and thigh regions should be palpated in a systematic fashion. The quadriceps, adductor, and hamstring muscle compartments of the thigh are palpated individually. The bony prominence of the proximal femur, the greater trochanter, is palpated. Direct palpation of the femoral neck and shaft is difficult because of overlying muscle and soft tissue. With fractures in this region, however, movement of fracture surfaces or crepitation often can be appreciated with gentle palpation. All areas of localized tenderness and swelling should be noted and an attempt made to correlate these areas with underlying anatomic structures.

Movements

In the absence of obvious deformity, an attempt should be made to gently move the hip joint. This can be accomplished most effectively by flexing the hip and knee joints simultaneously. Rotation of the hip also can be assessed with the extremity in this position. Significant pain with these maneuvers or limitation of movement is a sign of significant musculoskeletal injury. With fracture of the femoral shaft a characteristic posterior sag of the thigh will be noted when the hip and knee are flexed. Nondisplaced fractures of the proximal femur may exhibit a complete, though painful, passive range of motion. Full passive range of motion of the hip without pain usually rules out a fracture or dislocation.

Neurovascular Examination

With injuries of the hip and thigh a focused neurologic assessment of the injured extremity is indicated because of the potential for peripheral nerve injury. Posterior hip dislocations can be associated with sciatic nerve palsy, and femoral shaft fractures can be associated with either femoral or sciatic nerve injury. It is critical that the neurologic status of the extremity be determined and documented before initiation of any treatments, which could themselves compromise the neurologic status of the limb. Both motor and sensory function should be assessed in the involved leg. Certain simple tests can be performed quickly to evaluate peripheral nerve function in the involved extremity. Abnormal findings in any one of these tests warrants a more detailed examination.

Femoral nerve

Motor: knee extension (quadriceps)

Sensory: medial malleolus of ankle (saphenous nerve)

Sciatic nerve

Motor: knee flexion (hamstrings)

Tibial nerve

Motor: ankle plantar flexion (gastrocnemius-soleus complex)

Sensory: plantar foot (medial and lateral plantar nerves)

Superficial peroneal nerve

Motor: ankle eversion (peroneal muscles)

Sensory: dorsum of foot

Deep peroneal nerve

Motor: great toe extension (extensor hallucis longus)

Sensory: first web space dorsum of foot

Understanding the anatomy of the peripheral nerves in the lower extremity is essential: The sciatic nerve branches into the tibial and common peroneal nerves just proximal to the knee. The common peroneal subsequently gives rise to superficial and deep branches below the knee. Thus sciatic nerve injury at the level of the hip or proximal thigh may present with a combination of peroneal and tibial nerve dysfunction in the lower leg. Most commonly the peroneal division is affected most severely. In fact, tibial nerve function may be normal in many cases of proximal sciatic nerve palsy.

The possibility of vascular injury in association with hip and thigh trauma also must be considered. This usually can be assessed quickly by palpation of the dorsalis pedis pulse on the dorsum of the foot or the posterior tibial pulse behind the medial malleolus of the ankle. Palpable distal pulses indicate adequate peripheral blood flow distal to the site of injury.

■ FURTHER ORDERS

All patients sustaining hip and thigh trauma should be referred for radiographs of the hip and femur. Standard screening radiographs for the hip consist of AP and cross table lateral views. The lateral image, although somewhat difficult to obtain, is essential for complete evaluation of a hip dislocation or proximal femur fracture. AP and lateral radiographs also should be obtained for suspected injury to the femoral shaft. A common mistake is to obtain a single set of AP and lateral images for the evaluation of the hip and femur. Standard AP and lateral radiographs of the femur usually do not afford adequate visualization of the hip and proximal femur. Therefore, if a hip dislocation or proximal femur fracture is suspected, separate radiographs of the hip must be obtained.

■ MANAGEMENT

If radiographs of the hip and femur are negative and soft tissue trauma is suspected (muscular injury), symptomatic treatment is indicated. The muscle group involved should be identified through physical examination. Cold therapy and NSAIDs should be administered to reduce inflammation and provide analgesia. Although these injuries can be quite painful, early motion of the hip and knee must be encouraged. This is particularly important in quadriceps contusions, in which early motion has been shown to reduce the incidence of posttraumatic heterotopic ossification. Patients also should be encouraged to continue full weight bearing on the involved extremity. In rare cases, proximal hamstring tendon avulsions require operative intervention.

In the patient with hip pain but negative initial radiographs of the hip and femur and no evidence of soft tissue trauma, orthopaedic consultation is appropriate to rule out an occult fracture of the proximal femur. These fractures are suspected in patients with significant pain and inability to bear weight following injury, despite negative screening radiographs. Additional radiographic studies (bone scan, CT scan, or MRI) usually are indicated to confirm or exclude fracture.

The immediate management of fractures of the hip and thigh should be directed toward ensuring adequate immobilization of the extremity. Immobilization provides pain relief and protects the extremity against further damage. In elderly patients with fractures of the proximal femur ("hip" fractures), this can be accomplished effectively with Buck's traction using 10 pounds of longitudinal traction (Fig. 29–1*B*). If the patient is in a Hare traction splint, every attempt should be made to remove this splint as soon as possible because of the potential for soft tissue complications. The most effective means of obtaining immobilization in patients with femoral shaft fractures is through longitudinal skeletal traction. The traction pin, which can be inserted in either the proximal tibia (most commonly) or distal femur, also can prove useful for intraoperative fracture reduction at the time of definitive fracture treatment. In general the decision to insert a skeletal traction pin should be made in consultation with the treating orthopaedist.

Immediate orthopaedic consultation is indicated for all hip dislocations and fractures of the femur (proximal femur and femoral shaft). Certain types of injuries, such as hip dislocations, femoral neck fractures in young patients, and open fractures, require emergent treatment to optimize outcome. Other injuries, such as hip fractures in the elderly patient, often can be treated on a more elective basis. As with all musculoskeletal injuries, the treatment recommended by the consulting orthopaedist will be based on the injury as well as on consideration of factors specific to the individual patient.

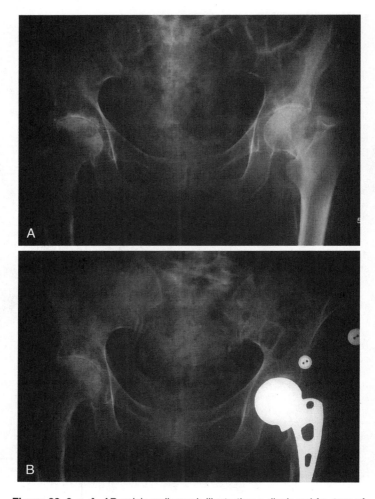

Figure 29–3 □ **A,** AP pelvic radiograph illustrating a displaced fracture of the left femoral neck. **B,** Postoperative AP pelvic radiograph demonstrating prosthetic replacement of the left proximal femur (hemiarthroplasty).

Hip dislocations are the result of high-energy trauma. Posterior dislocations of the hip, which are much more common than anterior dislocations, are associated with a significant risk of damage to the femoral head blood supply. Interference with the blood supply can result in irreversible osteonecrosis of the femoral head. For this reason, emergent reduction of the hip is indicated in all cases. Sig-

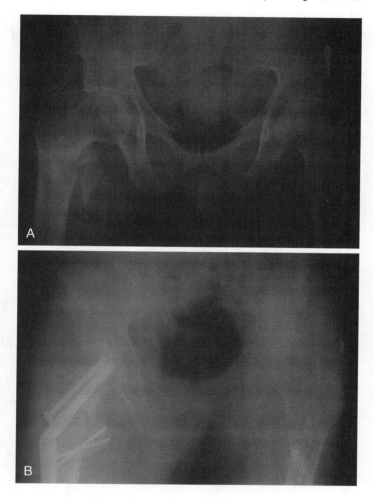

Figure 29–4 □ **A,** AP pelvic radiograph illustrating a displaced intertrochanteric fracture of the right proximal femur. **B,** Postoperative radiograph demonstrating reduction and internal fixation of the right intertrochanteric femur fracture.

nificant force is necessary to reduce a dislocated hip. In most cases, however, reduction can be accomplished with closed techniques and appropriate sedation. A dislocated hip should be reduced within 6 to 8 hours of the injury, and the reduction should not be delayed in favor of lower priority diagnostic procedures. Following reduction a CT scan of the affected hip is indicated to rule out femoral head fracture, associated posterior wall acetabular fracture, or intraarticular bone fragments.

A displaced fracture of the femoral neck in a young patient, although rare, also represents a surgical emergency. Prolonged fracture displacement is associated with a high risk of nonunion and femoral head osteonecrosis. Urgent anatomic fracture reduction and stabilization afford the best chance of a successful outcome. Fractures of the femoral head also may require operative reduction and fixation, depending on the fracture location, size of fragment(s), and degree of displacement.

"Hip fracture" in the elderly patient most commonly refers to fracture of the femoral neck or intertrochanteric region of the proximal femur. In contrast to proximal femoral fractures in young patients, these injuries characteristically are the result of low-energy trauma and involve injury to osteoporotic bone. Although operative intervention usually is necessary, many of these injuries can be

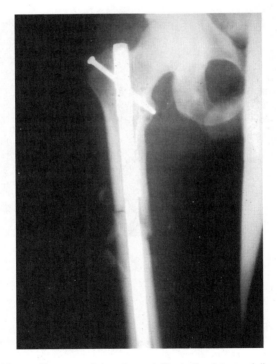

Figure 29–5 □ Postoperative radiograph illustrating intramedullary nail fixation of a femoral shaft fracture.

treated on a semielective basis. The treatment of femoral neck fractures in older patients generally is based on the degree of displacement. If the fracture is displaced minimally or is nondisplaced, closed reduction and percutaneous fixation is favored. On the other hand, if the fracture is displaced, prosthetic replacement of the proximal femur (hemiarthroplasty) commonly is performed (Fig. 29–3). Intertrochanteric femur fractures are managed best with surgical reduction and internal fixation (Fig. 29–4). The risk of nonunion and osteonecrosis is low with this fracture type, and semielective management is appropriate.

Fractures of the femoral diaphysis, including the subtrochanteric region, are best managed operatively in adults. Intramedullary fixation (IM nail) is used most often (Fig. 29–5), although plate fixation is sometimes indicated. The treatment of femoral shaft fractures generally is associated with excellent fracture healing and return of function. An attempt is made in these fractures to obtain skeletal stabilization within 24 hours of injury.

Open fractures require emergent orthopaedic intervention because of the relatively high risk of infection. Patients with open fractures require emergent operative debridement and appropriate skeletal stabilization. Any open wounds should be covered with a sterile povidone-iodine (Betadine)-soaked gauze dressing pending definitive operative management.

If compartment syndrome of the thigh is suspected on the basis of the injury mechanism and physical examination, emergent orthopaedic consultation is necessary. A compartment syndrome must be treated with emergent fasciotomy. Compartment syndromes are discussed in more detail in Chapter 32.

30

KNEE PAIN

C. Michael LeCroy

Injuries to the knee range widely in severity from simple sprains to complex intraarticular fractures. In contrast to other regions of the lower extremity, significant knee injuries occur frequently with both low- and high-energy mechanisms. In fact, knee pain is perhaps the most common musculoskeletal complaint following recreational injury. Most patients presenting for evaluation of knee pain will have a history of specific antecedent trauma. In contrast to the spine, pelvis, and hip, the knee is readily accessible for examination. This frequently allows the careful examiner to establish an accurate diagnosis through history and physical examination alone.

■ PHONE CALL

Questions

1. **How was the knee injured?**

   An understanding of the mechanism of injury is critical in the evaluation of musculoskeletal trauma. This is the initial step in the formulation of a differential diagnosis.

2. **Is there gross deformity?**

   Obvious deformity of the knee usually indicates fracture or dislocation or both.

3. **Is there swelling?**

   Swelling apparent almost immediately after the injury is a sign of significant bone or soft tissue trauma.

4. **Can the patient localize the pain to a specific area?**

   The ability of the patient to localize the pain to a specific region of the knee can be very helpful in establishing a diagnosis.

5. **Is there an associated skin wound or laceration?**

   An open wound should alert the physician to the potential for an open fracture or intraarticular communication. These conditions require urgent evaluation and treatment.

6. **Can the patient move the ipsilateral foot and toes?**

   Spontaneous or voluntary movements of the ipsilateral foot and toes distal to the site of injury can provide a rough assessment of whether there is concomitant neurologic injury. This must be evaluated subsequently by physical examination.

7. **Does the patient have a palpable distal pulse?**

   A palpable distal pulse can establish that blood flow is adequate distal to the site of injury. Although this does not rule out associated vascular trauma, it does signify sufficient peripheral circulation.

8. **Can the patient ambulate on the injured leg?**

   A history of weight bearing on the injured leg makes a significant fracture or dislocation of the knee highly unlikely.

9. **Are there any additional injuries?**

   As with all trauma to the musculoskeletal system, associated injuries to other body systems must be ruled out. This is particularly important in cases of high-energy trauma, in which the incidence of associated injuries is high.

10. **Is the patient hemodynamically stable?**

    Hemodynamic stability is the first priority of management in all trauma victims. If the patient is not hemodynamically stable, attention should be turned to the ABCs (airway, breathing, circulation) before the musculoskeletal injury is evaluated.

Orders

1. Ask the RN to immobilize the knee, particularly if evaluation of the patient is going to be delayed for any length of time. Immobilization will provide pain relief and prevent further soft tissue trauma. The knee can be immobilized easily with a commercial knee immobilizer. If such a device is not available, the knee can be immobilized effectively with wooden or plaster splints applied to the medial and lateral aspects of the extremity. Care should be taken to avoid constricting the extremity with tight circumferential straps or bandages.

2. If the patient has sustained a high-energy mechanism of injury, such as a motor vehicle accident, ask the RN to obtain immediate consultation with a trauma specialist (emergency medicine physician or general surgeon).

Inform RN

"I will arrive at the bedside within 30 minutes."

Recreational injuries to the knee rarely are limb threatening and generally do not require emergent evaluation. If open fracture or dislocation is suspected from the described injury mechanism and history, however, urgent evaluation is indicated. A delay in the diagnosis of popliteal artery injury in association with a knee dislocation can lead to loss of the extremity. In general, to minimize patient discomfort and optimize outcome, all injuries to the knee should be evaluated as soon as possible.

■ ELEVATOR THOUGHTS

Strains
- Distal quadriceps muscle strain or contusion

Sprains
- Medial collateral ligament injury
- Lateral collateral ligament injury

Dislocations
- Knee dislocation

Fractures
- Distal femoral fracture (Fig. 30–1)
  - Supracondylar
  - Intercondylar
- Patella fracture
- Tibial plateau fracture
- Tibial spine fracture
- Tibial tubercle fracture

Internal Derangements of Knee
- Chondral or osteochondral fracture
- Medial meniscus tear
- Lateral meniscus tear
- Anterior cruciate ligament tear
- Posterior cruciate ligament tear

Other
- Quadriceps tendon rupture
- Patellar tendon rupture
- Gastrocnemius avulsion

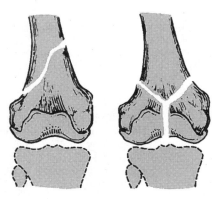

Figure 30–1 □ Supracondylar vs. intercondylar fractures of the distal femur. (From Browner BD, Jupiter JB, Levine AM, Trafton PG: Skeletal Trauma. Philadelphia, WB Saunders, 1992, p 1648.)

■ BEDSIDE

Vital Signs

A complete set of vital signs must be obtained in any trauma victim. In general, injury to the knee should not compromise the vital signs. As with trauma to other regions of the body, it should be expected that pain and anxiety will elevate the heart rate and blood pressure.

Selective History

How exactly was the knee injured?

Following preliminary assessment of the patient and once hemodynamic stability has been assured, the examiner should attempt to elicit as much information as possible regarding the mechanism of injury. This history ideally should include not only the forces involved but also the position of the extremity at the time of injury. In many cases an understanding of how the injury occurred can lead to an anatomic diagnosis. An important initial distinction with respect to knee injuries concerns whether high- or low-energy forces were involved (e.g., motor vehicle crash vs. recreational soccer injury). Victims of high-energy trauma to the knee are more likely to sustain a fracture or dislocation, whereas patients with low-energy trauma more often experience meniscus or ligament injuries. A history of a direct blow to the anterior aspect of the knee (e.g., dashboard injury) suggests a patella fracture or knee dislocation. Likewise, a history of blunt trauma to the medial or lateral aspects of the knee indicates lateral or medial collateral ligament injury, respectively. The patient may describe a twisting injury to the knee—a history often seen in meniscus injuries. A history of sudden deceleration with the foot planted strongly suggests anterior cruciate ligament injury. A history of an audible "pop" indicates an extensor mechanism disruption (quadriceps or patellar tendon rupture).

What was the condition of the patient immediately following the injury?

Knowing the patient's condition immediately following the accident or injury is helpful to the treating physician in assessing the potential for significant injury to the knee. For example, it is useful to determine whether the patient was able to ambulate at the scene. A patient who was ambulatory after injury is unlikely to have a fracture or dislocation. On the other hand, a history of immediate knee swelling (effusion) following injury strongly suggests significant intraarticular injury.

Can the patient localize the pain?

The patient should be asked to localize the pain. Patients with intraarticular fractures or cruciate ligament injuries usually will exhibit diffuse pain. In contrast, patients with collateral ligament or meniscus injuries often will localize their pain to either the medial or lateral aspects of the knee. Similarly, patients with patella fractures or extensor mechanism injuries often will note discomfort specifically in the anterior aspect of the knee. The patient also should be questioned regarding numbness or tingling in the affected lower extremity—symptoms that suggest a neurovascular injury.

What are the patient-specific factors?

A final category of information that must be elicited during this portion of the evaluation includes factors specific to the individual patient. The patient's age, occupation, and functional demands should be determined, as well as the existence of any comorbid factors and chronic medical conditions. Any history of prior knee injury or knee surgery also should be identified, so that acute trauma can be distinguished from preexisting conditions. This is a particular problem in the evaluation of knee trauma because of the prevalence of injuries to this joint. Although these patient-specific factors usually will not establish the diagnosis, they are useful in formulating a treatment plan and prognosis once the diagnosis has been made.

Selective Physical Examination

Inspection

The patient should be lying supine on a stretcher or hospital bed with both lower extremities exposed to above the knee. The degree of discomfort the patient is experiencing usually can be determined simply by observing the patient from the foot of the bed for a few seconds. This information may assist the examiner in determining the potential for significant fracture, dislocation, or ligament injury. Any swelling, ecchymosis, or deformity should be noted. With a knee dislocation, obvious incongruity of the femoral-tibial articulation usually is apparent; with other injuries, however, the physical findings are more subtle. Injuries to the knee often are appreciated best through comparison to the contralateral uninjured lower extremity. The injured knee also should be carefully inspected for any disruption of skin integrity. The communication of any wounds or lacerations with underlying fracture or articular surfaces must be ruled out. Finally, the patient should be observed for any spontaneous movement of the ipsilateral lower leg; such movement generally indicates intact neurovascular status.

Palpation

In contrast to the pelvis and hip, the knee is amenable to palpation. The knee should be palpated in a systematic fashion. All areas of localized tenderness and swelling should be noted and correlated with the underlying anatomic structures. The suprapatellar region should be palpated initially, followed by the knee joint itself, for an effusion. An effusion noted immediately after an injury usually indicates significant intraarticular injury. The contours of the distal femur, proximal tibia, and patella should be palpated directly. With fractures in this region, movement of the fracture surfaces or crepitation often can be appreciated through gentle palpation. The position of the patella relative to the underlying distal femur and proximal tibia should be determined. In disruption of the quadriceps tendon, the patella will be displaced distally, whereas in rupture of the patellar tendon the patella will be displaced proximally. The defect in the extensor mechanism often can be palpated directly in these injuries. The medial and lateral joint lines should be palpated next, followed by the medial and lateral collateral ligaments. Palpation of the joint line and collateral ligaments is facilitated by flexing the knee to 90 degrees.

Movements

An attempt should be made to gently move the knee. This is accomplished most effectively with the patient lying supine. Significant pain with this maneuver or limitation of movement is a sign of musculoskeletal injury. The range of movement allowed by the patient can be helpful in determining the type of injury incurred. For example, a fixed flexion contracture may indicate a meniscus tear. Patients with knee dislocation also will exhibit markedly restricted motion. Conversely, normal range of motion usually rules out significant fracture or dislocation about the knee. Finally, it is important to note that patients with internal derangements of the knee may present with near normal, although painful, range of motion.

If disruption of the extensor mechanism is suspected (patella fracture, quadriceps tendon rupture, or patellar tendon rupture), active extension of the knee also should be assessed. Inability to extend the flexed knee or to maintain knee extension corroborates an extensor mechanism injury.

Once the range of movement has been determined, the integrity of the collateral ligaments should be assessed. This is accomplished most effectively with the patient supine and the knee flexed 30 degrees, a position that eliminates the contribution of the cruciate ligaments to coronal plane stability of the knee joint. Varus stress is applied to the knee to test the lateral collateral ligament, and valgus stress to test the medial collateral ligament. Significant pain and joint space opening with these maneuvers indicate collateral ligament injury.

Special Tests for Internal Derangements of the Knee

In addition to observation, palpation, and assessment of range of motion, a complete examination of the knee following injury requires special maneuvers for determination of meniscus or cruciate ligament injury. It is important to emphasize that all the following tests should be performed on the injured knee as well as the uninjured contralateral knee whenever possible. This will allow for the appreciation of subtle differences and increase the sensitivity of the maneuvers.

McMurray's Test (Fig. 30–2).   This maneuver is performed by slowly extending the flexed knee with the leg externally rotated and with valgus stress to the knee joint. Pain and a palpable or audible click along the medial joint line indicate a tear of the posterior horn of the medial meniscus.

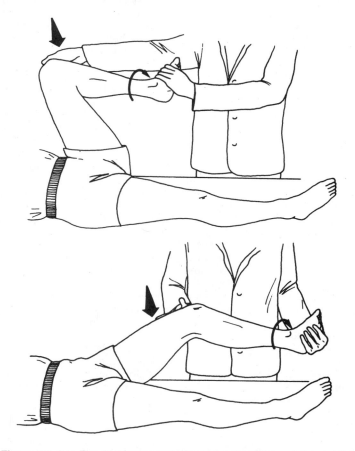

Figure 30–2 □ The McMurray test for diagnosis of tear of the medial meniscus. (From Birnbaum JS: The Musculoskeletal Manual, 2nd ed. Philadelphia, WB Saunders, 1986, p 181.)

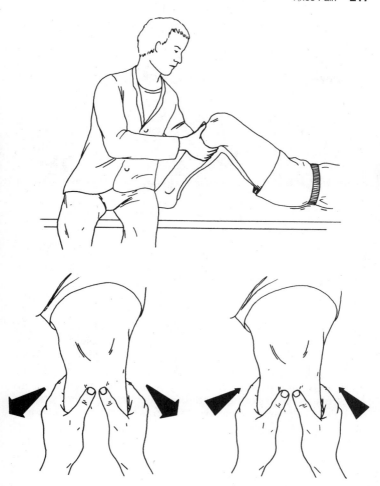

ANTERIOR DRAWER TEST
(for the ANTERIOR CRUCIATE LIGAMENT).

POSTERIOR DRAWER TEST
(for the POSTERIOR CRUCIATE LIGAMENT).

Figure 30–3 □ The anterior and posterior drawer tests for diagnosis of tears of the anterior and posterior cruciate ligaments, respectively. (From Birnbaum JS: The Musculoskeletal Manual, 2nd ed. Philadelphia, WB Saunders, 1986, p 179.)

Drawer Tests (Fig. 30–3). The anterior and posterior drawer tests are performed to identify injury to the anterior and posterior cruciate ligaments respectively. Both tests are performed with the patient supine and the knee flexed 90 degrees. With the patient's foot stabilized on the examining table, an attempt is made to dis-

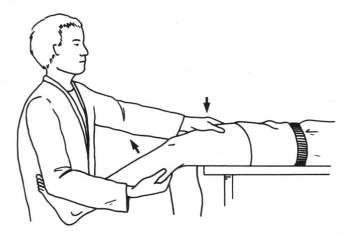

Figure 30–4 □ The Lachman test for diagnosis of anterior cruciate ligament injury. (From Birnbaum JS: The Musculoskeletal Manual, 2nd ed. Philadelphia, WB Saunders, 1986, p 180.)

place the tibia relative to the femur, first anteriorly (anterior drawer) and then posteriorly (posterior drawer). Significant displacement of the tibia indicates cruciate ligament injury.

Lachman's Test (Fig. 30–4). The Lachman test is said to be the most sensitive for the diagnosis of anterior cruciate ligament injury. This test is performed with the patient lying supine and the knee flexed 20 degrees. The distal femur is stabilized by the examiner's upper hand, and an anterior force is applied to the posterior aspect of the proximal tibia by the lower hand. Anterior translation of the tibia on the femur is measured. In an anterior cruciate–deficient knee, the tibia can be translated anteriorly for several millimeters without definite endpoint.

Pivot Shift Test (Fig. 30–5). This test also is performed with the patient lying supine. An internal rotation force to the leg and a valgus force to the knee are applied while the knee is taken from full extension into flexion. In anterior cruciate–deficient knees the examiner may be able to appreciate a "shift," representing reduction of the anteriorly displaced tibia relative to the femur.

Quadriceps Active Test. This test is the most sensitive for the diagnosis of posterior cruciate ligament insufficiency. The patient lies supine with the knee flexed 90 degrees. The examiner stabilizes the patient's foot to the examining table, and the patient is asked to attempt extension of the knee. In posterior cruciate–deficient knees the tibia will be observed to move anteriorly to a reduced position relative to the distal femur.

Neurovascular Examination

A focused neurologic assessment of the injured extremity is necessary in the patient with knee trauma because of the potential for neurologic injury following fractures and dislocation of the knee. The tibial branch of the sciatic nerve, the peroneal branch, or both branches may be injured. The extent of neurologic deficit depends primarily on the severity, as well as the level, of the injury. It therefore is critical to assess the integrity of motor and sensory functions for the tibial, superficial peroneal, and deep peroneal nerves in the lower leg. This can be accomplished with the simple tests described in Chapter 29 for quick assessment of peripheral nerve function in the lower extremity.

Vascular injury also may occur in fractures of the distal femur or in dislocations of the knee. Because vascular trauma is relatively common in these injuries and because the consequences of a missed diagnosis are devastating, it is incumbent on the examiner

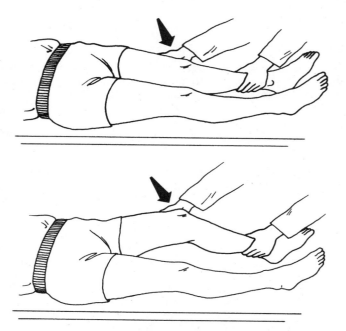

Figure 30–5 □ The pivot shift test for diagnosis of anterior cruciate ligament injury. (From Birnbaum JS: The Musculoskeletal Manual, 2nd ed. Philadelphia, WB Saunders, 1986, p 180.)

to rule out vascular compromise. The distal pulses should be palpated carefully; it is important to remember, however, that palpable distal pulses do not necessarily rule out vascular injury. If vascular injury is suspected, early consultation with a general or vascular surgeon is indicated, and arteriography of the affected extremity may be performed.

■ **FURTHER ORDERS**

All patients sustaining knee trauma should be referred for radiographs of the knee. Standard screening radiographs for the knee consist of AP and lateral views. Even with severe fracture or dislocation, it usually is possible to position the extremity for these two orthogonal images. Although most fractures of the knee region can be diagnosed on the AP and lateral images alone, additional plain radiographic views occasionally are indicated: The notch view may be helpful in the diagnosis of tibial spine fractures, and Merchant's (sunrise) view may be useful in the characterization of fractures of the distal femur or patella.

■ **MANAGEMENT**

Knee injuries are encountered commonly as a result of both high- and low-energy mechanisms. In general, the high-energy mechanisms usually cause fractures or dislocations, whereas the low-energy mechanisms cause soft tissue injuries (meniscus, ligament, or cartilage damage). The focus of the initial evaluation of the patient with knee pain due to injury should be to determine which of these types of injury the patient has sustained. Immediate orthopaedic consultation is indicated for all fractures of the distal femur, proximal tibia, and patella and for dislocation of the knee. On the other hand, soft tissue injuries and internal derangements of the knee often are managed most appropriately by a nonorthopaedist initially and subsequently are referred for orthopaedic follow-up.

Dislocation of the knee (Fig. 30–6) is an orthopaedic and general surgical emergency because of the high incidence of concomitant injury to the popliteal artery with the potential for compromise of limb vascularity. The knee dislocation should be reduced as soon as possible. This usually is not difficult; however, the knee often will subluxate or redislocate because of associated ligament injury. For this reason, it is wise to temporarily splint the knee following reduction while awaiting definitive treatment. Careful assessment of limb vascularity, often including arteriography, is essential in patients with knee dislocation. The decision whether to perform

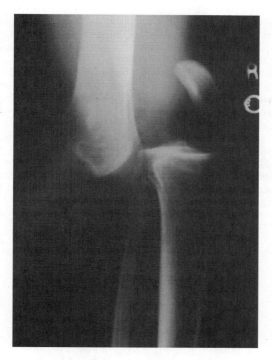

Figure 30–6 □ Lateral radiograph illustrating anterior dislocation of the knee joint.

the knee reduction and vascular assessment in the operating room is made by the consulting orthopaedic and general surgeons.

Supracondylar and intercondylar fractures of the distal femur are complex fractures that usually require operative management. If the fracture is nondisplaced, nonoperative treatment may be elected in certain patients (e.g., elderly, low demand). Most distal femoral fractures, however, are displaced and are managed best with operative reduction and fixation. An attempt is made to anatomically reduce an intraarticular extension of a fracture. A variety of intramedullary and extramedullary implants are available for stabilization of the distal femur to the femoral shaft.

Fractures of the tibial plateau are more common than fractures of the distal femur. The treatment of these injuries is based on the fracture pattern, the amount of articular surface displacement, and the functional demands of the patient. Nonoperative management with immobilization of the knee and protected weight bearing may be appropriate for simple fracture patterns with minimal displacement. As with periarticular fractures in other regions of the body, operative reduction and stabilization generally is indicated for fracture patterns with significant comminution or displacement of the articular surface.

Fractures of the tibial spine or tibial tubercle represent a subset of fractures of the proximal tibia; these injuries usually are a manifestation of avulsion of the anterior cruciate ligament or patellar tendon, respectively. The treatment of these injuries is based on the size of the avulsed bone fragment and the amount of displacement. Operative reduction and fixation are favored for large fragments with significant displacement.

Like other fractures of the knee region, fractures of the patella are characteristically the result of high-energy trauma (Fig. 30–7). The treatment of patella fractures is based on the amount of articular surface displacement as well as the integrity of the extensor mechanism of the knee. Nonoperative management is appropriate

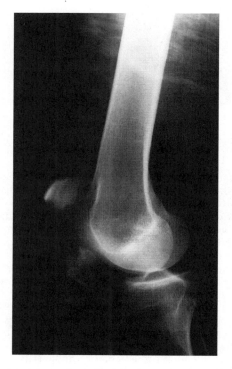

Figure 30–7 □ Lateral radiograph of the knee demonstrating a displaced fracture of the patella.

for minimally displaced fractures with intact active knee extension; otherwise, operative reduction and fixation are favored.

For open fractures, emergent orthopaedic intervention is indicated because of the significantly increased risk of infection. Patients with open fractures will require emergent operative debridement in addition to appropriate skeletal stabilization. Any open wounds should be covered with a sterile povidone-iodine (Betadine)-soaked gauze dressing pending definitive operative management.

Early orthopaedic consultation is indicated for disruptions of the extensor mechanism of the knee (quadriceps tendon or patellar tendon rupture). These injuries usually are treated with surgical repair on a semielective basis, and a favorable prognosis is expected unless the diagnosis or appropriate intervention is delayed. The patient is managed with a knee immobilizer, elevation of the extremity, and analgesic medication while awaiting definitive treatment.

If radiographs of the knee are negative and there is an intraarticular effusion, internal derangement of the knee should be suspected. The special physical examination maneuvers described earlier should be performed in an attempt to differentiate between meniscus, cruciate ligament, and cartilage injury. Symptomatic treatment alone is the usual initial management in these injuries. Consideration should be given to performing knee aspiration under sterile conditions in patients with tense effusions. Often several hundred milliliters of fluid can be aspirated from the joint, significantly relieving the pain. This procedure may be combined with infiltration of the knee joint with a short-acting anesthetic solution (e.g., 15 ml 1% lidocaine) to allow more accurate diagnostic examination of the knee. Other forms of acute management for internal derangements of the knee include application of a knee immobilizer, NSAIDs, and crutches for protected weight bearing. Outpatient orthopaedic follow-up should be arranged within 5 to 7 days of the injury. Orthopaedic follow-up may be indicated sooner in cases of fixed knee contracture with suspected incarcerated meniscus tear.

If radiographs of the knee are negative, if there is no significant effusion, and if extraarticular soft tissue trauma is suspected, symptomatic treatment is indicated. Cold therapy and NSAIDs should be administered to reduce inflammation and provide analgesia. Collateral ligament injuries should be managed with application of a knee immobilizer and orthopaedic follow-up within 7 to 10 days. If distal quadriceps contusion is suspected, early active knee motion should be encouraged to reduce the potential for posttraumatic heterotopic ossification. All patients with extraarticular soft tissue trauma should be encouraged to continue full weight bearing on the involved extremity.

31

LEG PAIN

C. Michael LeCroy

The leg is defined as the portion of the lower limb between the knee and ankle joints. Included within this region of the lower extremity are the tibia and fibula, the four muscle compartments of the leg, and the neurovascular structures that pass from the thigh to the foot. Pain in the leg is rare in the absence of trauma, and high-energy injury patterns are seen frequently following blunt trauma to the leg. The leg is particularly susceptible to bone injury because of the relatively subcutaneous position of the tibia anteriorly and medially. The leg is also the most common site of compartment syndrome. When trauma is experienced, the diagnosis usually is readily apparent following a thorough physical examination. This is due to the relatively straightforward anatomy in this region of the limb and to the accessibility of the anatomic structures to examination.

■ PHONE CALL

Questions

1. **How was the leg injured?**
   An understanding of the mechanism of injury is critical in the evaluation of musculoskeletal trauma. This is the initial step in the formulation of a differential diagnosis.
2. **Is there gross deformity?**
   Obvious deformity of the leg usually indicates fracture.
3. **Is there swelling?**
   Swelling apparent almost immediately after the injury is a sign of significant bone or soft tissue trauma.
4. **Can the patient localize the pain to a specific area?**
   The ability of the patient to localize the pain to a specific region of the leg can be very helpful in establishing a diagnosis.
5. **Is there an associated skin wound or laceration?**
   An open wound should alert the physician to the potential for an open fracture, a condition that requires urgent evaluation and treatment.
6. **Can the patient move the foot and toes of the injured leg?**
   Spontaneous or voluntary movements of the ipsilateral foot and toes distal to the site of injury can provide a rough assessment of whether there is concomitant neurologic injury. This must be evaluated subsequently by physical examination.

7. **Is there a palpable distal pulse?**

   A palpable distal pulse can establish that blood flow is adequate distal to the site of injury. Although this does not rule out associated vascular trauma, it does signify sufficient peripheral circulation.

8. **Can the patient ambulate on the injured leg?**

   A history of weight bearing on the injured leg makes a significant fracture of the leg highly unlikely.

9. **Does the patient have any additional injuries?**

   As with all trauma to the musculoskeletal system, associated injuries to other body systems must be ruled out. This is particularly important in cases of high-energy trauma, in which the incidence of associated injuries is high.

10. **Is the patient hemodynamically stable?**

    Hemodynamic stability is the first priority of management in all trauma victims. If the patient is not hemodynamically stable, attention should be turned to the ABCs (airway, breathing, circulation) before the musculoskeletal injury is evaluated.

Orders

1. Ask the RN to immobilize the leg, particularly if evaluation of the patient is going to be delayed. This will provide pain relief and will protect the extremity against further soft tissue injury. The leg and ankle may be immobilized with a provisional splint. It should be noted that effective immobilization of the leg cannot be achieved without including the ankle joint. Plaster or wooden splints commonly are used for this purpose; prefabricated splints also are available commercially. Care should be taken not to constrict the extremity with tight circumferential straps or bandages.

2. If the patient has sustained a high-energy mechanism of injury, such as a motor vehicle accident, ask the RN to obtain immediate consultation with a trauma specialist (emergency medicine physician or general surgeon).

Inform RN

"I will arrive at the bedside within 30 minutes."

Injuries to the leg can be limb threatening and should be evaluated on an urgent basis. If open fracture is suspected from the history, immediate evaluation is indicated. Also, the potential for compartment syndrome following blunt trauma to the leg, even in the absence of fracture, mandates urgent evaluation. In general, to optimize outcome and minimize patient discomfort, all injuries to the leg should be evaluated as soon as possible.

■ ELEVATOR THOUGHTS

- Strains
    - Anterior compartment muscle strain or contusion
    - Gastrocnemius strain or contusion
- Sprains
    - None
- Dislocations
    - None
- Fractures
    - Tibial shaft fracture
    - Fibular shaft fracture
- Other
    - Compartment syndrome of leg

■ BEDSIDE

Vital Signs

A complete set of vital signs should be obtained in any trauma patient. In general, an injury to the leg does not compromise the vital signs. As with trauma to other body regions, however, it should be expected that pain and anxiety will elevate the blood pressure and heart rate.

Selective History

How exactly was the leg injured?

Once the preliminary assessment is completed and hemodynamic stability has been assured, the examiner should attempt to obtain a more detailed description of the mechanism of injury. Most injuries to the leg involve direct, blunt trauma. Often an understanding of exactly how the injury occurred can lead to an anatomic diagnosis. One key variable involves the amount of energy involved in the injury. It can be expected that high-energy mechanisms, such as pedestrians struck by motor vehicles, will be associated with significantly more bone comminution, more soft tissue trauma, and an increased risk of compartment syndrome. The injury pattern usually is less severe following low-energy trauma.

What was the condition of the patient immediately following the injury?

It is also helpful to determine the condition of the patient immediately following the accident or injury. This information is quite useful in determining the potential for significant bone or soft tissue injury to the leg. A particular point of interest is whether the patient was able to ambulate at the scene, as a history of ambulation after injury usually rules out a tibial shaft fracture.

Can the patient localize the pain?

The patient should be asked to localize the pain in the leg if the site of injury is not immediately apparent (such as with an open fracture or an obvious fracture deformity). Patients with muscle strains or contusions will present with diffuse pain and tenderness, whereas patients with fracture of the tibial or fibular shaft or both usually will localize their pain precisely. The patient also should be questioned regarding numbness or tingling in the affected lower extremity—symptoms that suggest neurovascular injury.

What are the patient-specific factors?

A final category of information that should be elicited during this portion of the evaluation includes factors specific to the individual patient. The patient's age, occupation, past medical history, and functional demands should be determined. These factors will influence the injury prognosis considerably, as well as the treatment plan. For example, a history of cigarette smoking significantly increases the risk of complications adversely affecting bone and soft tissue healing. Any history of prior leg pain or trauma must be identified so that the acute injury can be distinguished from preexisting conditions.

Selective Physical Examination

Inspection

The patient should be lying supine on a hospital bed or stretcher with both lower extremities completely exposed. To begin the examination, it is helpful to observe the patient briefly from the foot of the bed to determine the degree of discomfort he or she is experiencing. This may assist the examiner in determining the potential for significant bone or soft tissue injury to the leg. Any swelling, ecchymosis, or deformity should be noted. Usually with fractures of the tibial shaft, deformity is readily apparent. With other injuries to the leg, however, the physical findings are more subtle. In determining the presence of deformity and swelling, it is often useful to compare the injured leg to the contralateral uninjured extremity. The entire injured leg should be inspected circumferentially for any disruption of skin integrity. The communication of any wounds or lacerations with underlying fracture must be ruled out. Finally, the patient should be observed for spontaneous movements of the ipsilateral foot and toes. Such movement usually indicates the neurovascular status of the extremity is intact.

Palpation

The leg should be palpated in a systematic fashion, beginning proximally and continuing distally to the level of the ankle joint. As mentioned, the tibia is particularly amenable to palpation because of its subcutaneous location. The entire medial subcutaneous border of the tibia may be palpated, and most fractures will be identified through this simple maneuver alone. The fibular shaft is more difficult to palpate, but it is accessible to deep palpation proximally and distally. Once the bones of the leg have been examined, the anterior, lateral, and posterior muscle compartments should be palpated individually. Significant circumferential swelling and pain with palpation should raise the index of suspicion for compartment syndrome of the leg.

Movements

If there is obvious deformity of the leg, such as that seen with a tibial shaft fracture, no attempt should be made to move the extremity. On the other hand, if bone injury is not immediately apparent, the leg should be elevated from the bed or stretcher and the ipsilateral knee and ankle joints sequentially flexed. It should be anticipated that these maneuvers will cause pain if there is muscle or bone injury of the leg because of the associated movement of muscle-tendon units during joint motion. Significant pain with these maneuvers or limitation of motion is a sign of musculoskeletal injury. In contrast, the absence of significant discomfort in the leg with ankle and knee motion usually rules out fracture or significant soft tissue injury.

Neurovascular Examination

A focused neurologic assessment of the injured extremity is necessary to exclude concomitant neurologic injury. With fractures and soft tissue injuries to the leg the common peroneal nerve is most at risk where it courses around the neck of the fibula proximally. An attempt should be made to verify the integrity of motor and sensory function for the superficial peroneal, deep peroneal, and tibial nerves in the leg and foot. This can be accomplished effectively using the tests described in Chapter 29 for assessment of peripheral nerve function in the lower extremity.

In contrast to fractures and dislocations about the knee, vascular injury is relatively rare with injuries to the leg. The trifurcation of the popliteal artery just below the knee usually ensures adequate blood flow to the distal extremity even with arterial disruption in one compartment. Nevertheless it is important to assess the adequacy of vascular flow to the ankle and foot distal to the injury by palpation of the posterior tibial and dorsalis pedis pulses. If one or both pulses cannot be directly palpated because of soft tissue swelling or relative hypotension, Doppler evaluation of the pulses is indicated. Early consultation with a general or vascular surgeon is indicated in the absence of distal pulses. The neurovascular status of the distal extremity should be closely monitored in the presence of actual or impending compartment syndrome of the leg, as discussed in Chapter 32.

■ FURTHER ORDERS

All patients sustaining an injury to the leg should be referred for radiographs. Standard screening radiographs for the leg consist of AP and lateral views of the involved tibia. These views will provide adequate visualization of the diaphyses of the tibia and fibula. If fracture is suspected proximally or distally, however, these views should be supplemented by AP and lateral radiographs of the knee or ankle respectively. With a tibial fracture it is often not possible to position the extremity adequately for images in the true coronal and sagittal planes; nevertheless an attempt should be made to obtain two orthogonal images for adequate fracture characterization.

■ MANAGEMENT

The immediate management of leg injury requires immobilization of the extremity to minimize patient discomfort and prevent further soft tissue trauma. A plaster splint is the most effective way to immobilize the leg. A standard "posterior splint," consisting of splints along the plantar foot and posterior calf, supplemented by a "sugar tong" splint across the ankle joint along the medial and lateral aspects of the leg will provide effective immobilization and maintain the ankle joint in neutral position. Prefabricated splints also are available in many hospitals. All splints should be well padded to accommodate the anticipated soft tissue swelling.

Immediate orthopaedic consultation is indicated for all fractures of the tibia and fibula. The optimum treatment for closed tibial shaft fractures is a topic of debate among orthopaedic surgeons. Fracture characteristics, patient-specific factors, and individual physician experience all play important roles in the determination of the most appropriate treatment. Isolated fractures of the tibial shaft with minimal displacement and comminution can be treated effectively using closed techniques with reduction (if necessary) and casting (Fig. 31–1). In general, acceptable reduction in the tibia requires less than 5 degrees angulation in the coronal plane and less than 10 degrees in the sagittal plane. If closed management is selected, care must be taken not to apply a circumferential cast acutely to a swollen extremity.

Tibial shaft fractures with significant displacement or comminution often are managed best by operative stabilization. Closed reduction with intramedullary nail fixation consistently yields good results in the treatment of such fractures (Fig. 31–2). Fractures involving the proximal or distal metaphyseal regions of the tibia often are treated surgically as well, either with intramedullary fixation or external fixation. Regardless of the treatment method selected, protected weight bearing is indicated initially for all fractures of the tibial shaft. Patients should be counseled that 4 to 6 months may be required for complete fracture healing.

Open fractures of the tibia represent a unique challenge. The extensive periosteal stripping and soft tissue damage associated with these injuries compromise the tenuous vascular supply to the bone, and bacterial contamination is common, placing the patient at high risk for healing complications and infection. Immediate orthopaedic consultation is indicated for these injuries, as urgent operative debridement and skeletal stabilization are necessary. Any open wounds should be covered with a sterile povidone-iodine (Betadine)-soaked gauze dressing pending definitive operative management. An attempt should be made to prevent iatrogenic contamination of such injuries by limiting the number of "looks" at the wound.

Fractures of the fibular shaft usually are seen in association with fractures of the tibia. The treatment for these injuries is dictated by the tibial shaft fracture pattern, as described above. Isolated fibular shaft fractures, when they do occur, are stable injuries and can

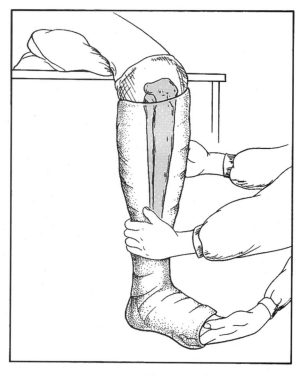

Figure 31–1 □ Closed reduction and cast immobilization of a tibial shaft fracture. (From Browner BD, Jupiter JB, Levine AM, Trafton PG: Skeletal Trauma. Philadelphia, WB Saunders, 1992, p 1804.)

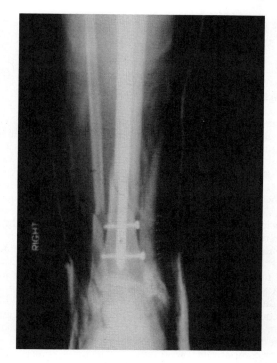

Figure 31–2 □ AP radiograph of the tibia illustrating intramedullary nail fixation of a tibial shaft fracture.

be treated symptomatically. A short period of splinting usually is indicated for comfort, followed by early mobilization and weight bearing. A short-leg walking cast may be used for 3 to 6 weeks in patients with significant discomfort. Healing complications are uncommon in these fractures.

As mentioned previously, the leg is the most common location for a compartment syndrome. If compartment syndrome is suspected on the basis of the mechanism of injury and physical examination, emergent orthopaedic consultation is necessary. A compartment syndrome must be treated with emergent fasciotomy. Compartment syndromes are discussed in more detail in Chapter 32.

If radiographs of the leg are negative and soft tissue trauma is suspected, symptomatic treatment is indicated. Cold therapy and NSAIDs should be administered acutely to reduce inflammation and provide analgesia. Splinting generally is not indicated, as this may actually delay recovery. Immediate motion of the knee and ankle joints should be encouraged, as well as continued full weight bearing on the involved extremity.

32

COMPARTMENT SYNDROME

C. Michael LeCroy

A compartment syndrome is a condition in which the circulation within a closed compartment is compromised by an increase in pressure within the compartment. A compartment syndrome can cause tissue ischemia and, if untreated, tissue death. Injury to neuromuscular structures can be irreversible, and extremity function may be severely compromised. The leading causes of compartment syndrome include fractures, blunt soft tissue trauma, arterial injury, limb compression, burns, and constricting dressings and splints or casts. The physician should understand that a compartment syndrome can be the result of the injury itself or of its treatment. The leg is by far the most common location for a compartment syndrome. The leg contains four well-defined compartments of muscle groups and their associated neurovascular structures. Other possible locations for compartment syndrome are the thigh (three compartments), the forearm (two compartments), the foot (four compartments), and the hand (many compartments). The key to the successful management of compartment syndrome is early recognition and institution of appropriate treatment. The physician must always be alert to the potential for compartment syndrome so that timely diagnosis can be made and irreversible tissue damage prevented.

■ PHONE CALL

Questions

1. **Which extremity is injured?**

    The physician first should attempt to identify which extremity is injured. A compartment syndrome is encountered most commonly in the lower extremity.

2. **What part of the extremity is injured?**

    The patient's ability to localize injury within the extremity can assist in determining the potential for a compartment syndrome. The most common location for a compartment syndrome is the leg.

3. **How did the injury occur?**

    An understanding of the mechanism of injury is critical in the evaluation of musculoskeletal trauma. This is the initial step in the formulation of a differential diagnosis. Particularly a history of high-energy blunt trauma, limb compression, or burn should alert the physician to the potential for compartment syndrome.

4. **Has the patient received any treatment for the injury (i.e., dressing, splint, or cast)?**

   A history of treatment for skeletal injury should alert the physician to the potential for compartment syndrome due to constricting dressings, splints, or casts.

5. **Is there gross deformity?**

   Obvious deformity of the extremity usually indicates fracture or dislocation or both.

6. **Is there swelling?**

   Swelling apparent almost immediately after injury is a sign of significant bone or soft tissue trauma. In addition, circumferential swelling of the extremity can be a sign of compartment syndrome.

7. **Is there an associated skin wound or laceration?**

   An open wound should alert the physician to the potential for an open fracture or arterial injury in the extremity. These conditions require urgent evaluation and treatment.

8. **Can the patient move the fingers or toes of the injured extremity?**

   Spontaneous or voluntary movement of the ipsilateral digits distal to the site of injury can provide a rough assessment of whether there is concomitant neurologic deficit. Paresis is a late finding in compartment syndrome.

9. **Does the patient complain of numbness or tingling in the fingers or toes of the injured extremity?**

   Complaints of numbness or paresthesias in the extremity following skeletal injury can be a sign of neurologic injury. As with paresis, these sensory disturbances are late findings in compartment syndrome.

10. **Does the patient have a distal pulse?**

    A palpable distal pulse can establish that blood flow is adequate distal to the site of injury. A palpable distal pulse, however, does not exclude the diagnosis of compartment syndrome.

11. **Does the patient have any additional injuries?**

    As with all trauma to the musculoskeletal system, associated injuries to other body systems must be ruled out. This is particularly important in cases of high-energy trauma, in which the incidence of associated injuries is high.

12. **Is the patient hemodynamically stable?**

    Hemodynamic stability is the first priority of management in all trauma victims. If the patient is not hemodynamically stable, attention should be turned to the ABCs (airway, breathing, circulation) before the musculoskeletal injury is evaluated.

Orders

1. Ask the RN to immobilize the injured extremity, particularly if a fracture is suspected from the mechanism of injury. This will re-

duce pain and prevent further soft tissue damage from bone fragments. See earlier chapters for techniques of immobilization.

2. If the patient already has been treated for the extremity injury, ask the RN to loosen or remove any circumferential dressings or splints. If a cast is in place, ask the RN to obtain the appropriate equipment for cast modification or removal.

3. Tell the RN *not* to elevate the injured extremity. In general, elevation of extremity injuries minimizes soft tissue swelling. In the presence of actual or impending compartment syndrome, however, elevation may actually worsen the condition by further diminishing arterial inflow.

4. If the patient has sustained a high-energy mechanism of injury, such as a motor vehicle accident, ask the RN to obtain immediate consultation with a trauma specialist (emergency medicine physician or general surgeon).

Inform RN

"I will arrive at the bedside immediately."

The successful management of compartment syndromes requires a high index of suspicion for its occurrence and careful evaluation of the patient. If compartment syndrome is suspected on the basis of the mechanism of injury and described symptoms, emergent evaluation is indicated.

■ ELEVATOR THOUGHTS

The differential diagnoses of injuries to the upper and lower extremities are covered in the other chapters of this section. In evaluating any extremity injury, all possible pertinent diagnoses should be kept firmly in mind. The physician must remember that compartment syndrome is associated with a variety of injuries to the extremities. The most important step in the successful management of a compartment syndrome is to recognize the potential for its occurrence. The next step is to understand the possible causes of the condition. The following section lists the potential locations of compartment syndromes, as well as factors that can contribute to the development of these syndromes.

Potential Locations of Compartment Syndrome
- Lower extremity
  Leg (most common)
  Thigh
  Foot
- Upper extremity
  Forearm
  Hand

Potential Causes of Compartment Syndrome
- Fracture
- Dislocation
- Blunt soft tissue trauma
- Arterial injury
- Limb compression
- Burns
- Constricting dressings, splints, or casts
- Severe hemorrhage (i.e., in hemophilia)

■ BEDSIDE

Vital Signs

A complete set of vital signs is essential in the evaluation of any trauma patient. A particularly important measurement in the evaluation of the patient with potential compartment syndrome is the diastolic blood pressure. The difference between the diastolic blood pressure and the measured compartment pressure can establish a definitive diagnosis of compartment syndrome; this is discussed in the Management portion of this chapter.

Selective History

How exactly did the injury occur?

The key to the successful management of a compartment syndrome is to maintain a high index of suspicion for its occurrence. The history of injury is the most important factor influencing this index of suspicion. Once the preliminary assessment has been completed and hemodynamic stability assured, the examiner should make every attempt to obtain a detailed description of the mechanism of injury. In general, compartment syndromes are more common following high-energy blunt trauma to an extremity. Examples of injuries in which compartment syndrome should be suspected include pedestrian vs. motor vehicle trauma and crushing injuries. If the patient is unable to provide details regarding the mechanism of injury, this information often can be obtained from emergency medical personnel or witnesses.

Has the patient sustained a penetrating injury to the extremity?

Another important potential cause of compartment syndrome is arterial disruption, which may occur with fracture, dislocation, or penetrating trauma to the extremity. Therefore it is important to elicit from the patient any history of penetrating injury to the extremity. Common penetrating injuries include gunshot wounds and stab wounds. A penetrating injury in conjunction with physical examination findings of arterial insufficiency should elevate the index of suspicion for a compartment syndrome.

Is there a history of burn injury or limb compression?

If fracture, blunt soft tissue trauma, and arterial disruption can be ruled out on the basis of the history, consideration should be given to other potential causes of compartment syndromes, such as burns and limb compression. Patients should be questioned for any history of burn injury, although in most cases this will be apparent from the initial assessment. Compartment syndrome can be caused by limb compression in patients who have remained in one position for a long time, usually following acute alcohol intoxication or drug overdose.

Has the patient undergone treatment for a musculoskeletal injury?

Compartment syndromes can be iatrogenic following treatment of musculoskeletal injuries. Circumferential constricting dressings, splints, or casts are usually implicated. If the patient being evaluated has been treated previously for an extremity injury, it is critical to identify the injury as well as the type of treatment rendered. A history of prior knee or elbow dislocation should increase suspicion for a compartment syndrome of the leg or forearm, respectively. Similarly, a history of vigorous closed reduction and plaster immobilization of an extremity or a history of prolonged use of a pneumatic tourniquet during an orthopaedic surgical procedure may be associated with an increased risk of compartment syndrome.

What are the patient-specific factors?

A final category of information that must be elicited during this portion of the evaluation includes factors specific to the individual patient. The patient's age, occupation, and functional demands should be determined, as well as any comorbid factors and chronic medical conditions. Although these patient-specific factors usually will not establish the diagnosis, they are quite useful in formulating a treatment plan and prognosis once the diagnosis has been made.

Selective Physical Examination

A thorough physical examination, along with a high index of suspicion, is critical to the successful diagnosis and management of compartment syndrome. In contrast to a fracture, where radiographs usually provide the diagnosis, the diagnosis of compartment syndrome is largely based on physical examination findings. In fact, it is fair to say that the diagnosis of a compartment syndrome cannot be established in the absence of swelling, pain, and the other physical findings described below. Finally, the physician should remember that a compartment syndrome is a dynamic, evolving process. This underscores the importance of frequent, serial examinations of the extremity at risk.

Inspection

The patient should be examined with the involved extremity completely exposed. Notation should be made of any swelling, skin discoloration, or deformity. Particular attention should be paid to the color of the digits distally in the extremity, as pallor suggests compromised vascular flow. The examiner also should attempt to determine the degree of discomfort the patient is experiencing by simply observing him or her from the foot of the bed for a few seconds. Patients with compartment syndrome characteristically will experience significant pain, often more than would be expected from the concomitant injuries. The extremity also should be inspected for any disruptions of skin integrity. It is important to remember that an open wound *does not* rule out a diagnosis of compartment syndrome. Compartment syndromes can and do occur with open fractures.

Palpation

The extremity should be palpated in a systematic fashion, taking care to palpate all bone prominences as well as all muscle compartments. Movement of fracture surfaces or crepitation often can be appreciated with gentle palpation. The physician should attempt to distinguish between localized areas of tenderness and swelling and diffuse tenderness and swelling. Compartment syndromes exhibit diffuse, prominent swelling of the involved portion of the extremity and exquisite, nonfocal tenderness to palpation. In most cases the pain with palpation is greater than would be expected from the concomitant injuries. It should be emphasized that although a diagnosis of compartment syndrome cannot be established in the absence of significant swelling, the physician should remember that every swollen extremity does not have a compartment syndrome. Swelling and pain with palpation are useful physical findings but alone do not establish a diagnosis of compartment syndrome.

Movements

An attempt should be made to gently move the joints of the involved extremity. Significant *pain with passive stretch* is the sine qua non of compartment syndrome. For example, in a compartment syndrome of the leg, intense pain is noted with passive dorsiflexion of the ankle and toes. In compartment syndrome of the forearm, significant pain is noted with passive flexion and extension of the wrist. Pain with passive stretch is an important factor in differentiating the limb with a compartment syndrome from other swollen and painful limbs. Although serial examinations are necessary, the absence of pain with passive stretch in the conscious patient can help rule out a diagnosis of compartment syndrome.

Neurovascular Examination

Careful evaluation of distal neurovascular function is critical in an extremity at risk for compartment syndrome. Distal pulses, digital sensation, and motor function should be assessed. Compartment syndrome compromises vascular inflow to the extremity and, in its later stages, causes neuromuscular damage. Thus, abnormal findings on neurovascular examination in a patient with a compartment syndrome are evidence of an advanced stage of the process. Pulselessness, paresthesias, and paresis (weakness) are all late signs of potentially irreversible tissue damage. Conversely, a normal neurovascular examination is reassuring but does not rule out an impending or actual compartment syndrome. The physician must rely on all the physical findings described above and repeatedly assess the extremity at risk.

Summary

A detailed, accurate physical examination is critical to the diagnosis of compartment syndrome. Since compartment syndrome is a dynamic process, the examination must be repeated on a serial basis in the extremity at risk. The following signs are useful to remember:

The Ps of Compartment Syndromes
- **Pain** with **passive** stretch
- **Pain** out of **proportion** to injury
- **Pressure** (swelling)
- **Pallor**
- **Pulselessness, paresthesias,** and **paresis** (all late findings)

■ FURTHER ORDERS

Complete screening radiographs of the involved extremity should be ordered for all patients under evaluation for compartment syndrome. The recommended radiographic images for extremity injuries are discussed in other chapters. In general, two orthogonal images should be obtained to allow the identification and characterization of potential skeletal injury. If distal pulses cannot be palpated in the involved extremity, Doppler examination should be performed.

■ MANAGEMENT

The successful management of a compartment syndrome begins with knowing the circumstances under which it can occur. The history of injury is critical in raising the suspicion of compartment syndrome. It should be suspected in any extremity that has sustained high-energy soft tissue or bone trauma, arterial disruption, a burn, or limb compression. The findings on serial physical examinations are used to confirm or exclude the diagnosis. The diagnosis of compartment syndrome is thus primarily a clinical one, and accurate diagnosis depends considerably on the experience and training of the examiner.

Immediate orthopaedic consultation should be obtained if compartment syndrome in an extremity is suspected. This is true even if radiographs of the extremity are negative, since compartment syndromes can occur in the absence of fracture or dislocation. The orthopaedic consultant will assist in determining the mechanism of injury, reviewing the radiographs, and evaluating the involved extremity. Time is of the essence in establishing the diagnosis and instituting the appropriate intervention.

The diagnosis of compartment syndrome relies heavily on certain physical findings in the conscious patient—particularly pain out of proportion to the injury and pain with passive movement of the extremity. It is important to recognize that these findings at times cannot be elicited in the unconscious, multiply injured, or head-injured patient. In these patients the physician must maintain an even higher index of suspicion for compartment syndrome and a lower threshold for further diagnostic or therapeutic interventions.

If a patient who previously has undergone treatment for an extremity injury is thought to have an impending compartment syndrome, it is imperative to remove or release tight dressings, splints, or casts. These patients will be noted to complain of intense pain out of proportion to that which is expected on the basis of their skeletal injury. Casts should be split and the cotton padding underneath divided as well. All circumferential dressings should be released to the level of the skin. If these measures are not sufficient to decrease symptoms and improve physical findings, the dressings or plaster or both should be removed entirely.

The most important variables in the diagnosis of compartment syndrome are the history of injury and the physical findings. The importance of direct monitoring of compartment pressures in the diagnosis of compartment syndrome is less clear and currently is under debate. Compartment pressure should not be measured without orthopaedic consultation. The decision to proceed with compartment pressure measurement should be made by the consulting surgeon after consideration of the history and physical findings. Compartment pressure measurements most commonly are obtained to corroborate a clinical diagnosis of compartment syndrome or to determine compartment pressures in patients with an unreliable physical examination (i.e., unconscious, head injured). How much weight should be given to compartment pressure measurements in excluding the diagnosis of compartment syndrome when physical findings are positive is less clear.

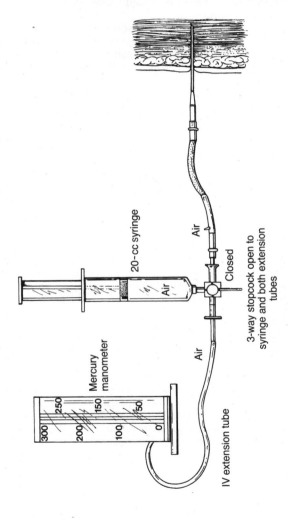

Figure 32–1 □ The Whitesides needle injection technique for compartment pressure measurement. (Redrawn from Whitesides T Jr. et al: Clin Orthop 113:46, 1975.)

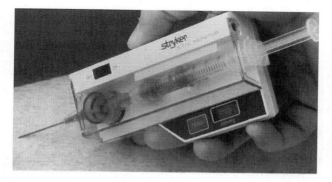

Figure 32–2 □ The Stic catheter for compartment pressure measurement. (Courtesy Stryker Mississauga, Ontario, Canada.)

Extremity compartment pressures can be determined with a variety of techniques, ranging from a simple arterial line setup to a needle injection manometer (Whitesides technique—Fig. 32–1). Most commonly compartment pressures are measured with commercially available hand-held monitors (Fig. 32–2). Continuous compartment pressure monitoring rarely is indicated.

There is considerable debate regarding the pressure threshold necessary to establish a diagnosis of compartment syndrome. Some authors have recommended intervention for pressures as low as 30 mm Hg, whereas others have suggested that pressures up to 45 mm Hg are acceptable before decompression is necessary. In recent years, evidence has supported the importance of the relationship between the measured compartment pressure and the patient's diastolic blood pressure. It has been suggested that a compartment pressure within 30 mm Hg of the patient's diastolic blood pressure is the most sensitive indicator of a true compartment syndrome.

Although the diagnosis of compartment syndrome rarely is clear-cut and requires considerable clinical experience and acumen, the treatment of a compartment syndrome is straightforward. Compartment syndromes must be treated surgically with decompressive fasciotomy of all involved compartments. All compartments must be released completely over their entire length. Several large incisions usually are required to accomplish this. Muscles are examined carefully for any necrotic tissue, which must be debrided if present. Wounds commonly are left open or loosely closed, with one or more return trips to the operating room expected. Following is a brief summary of the incisions required to treat compartment syndromes in the extremities:

- **Leg:** two incisions generally preferred, one medial and one lateral, for decompression of all four compartments (Fig. 32–3)

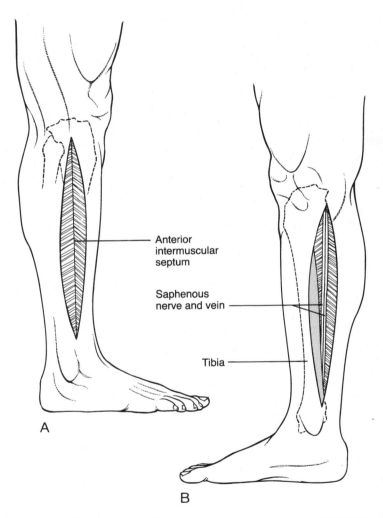

Anterior
intermuscular
septum

Saphenous
nerve and vein

Tibia

A

B

Figure 32–3 □ The two-incision technique for decompressive fasciotomy of the leg. Medial and lateral incisions are necessary to adequately release all four compartments of the leg. (Redrawn from AAOS Instructional Course Lectures, vol 32. St Louis, CV Mosby, 1983, pp 519–520.)

- **Thigh:** one or two incisions required, depending on the number of compartments involved (quadriceps, hamstring, or adductor muscle groups)
- **Foot:** two or three incisions usually required on the dorsal and medial surfaces
- **Forearm:** two incisions required, one dorsal for the extensor compartment, and one volar for the flexor compartment
- **Hand:** two or three incisions required for decompression of the intrinsic muscles, usually dorsally with or without a radial incision in the palm for the thenar muscle group; a separate volar incision for release of the median nerve in the carpal tunnel also may be required

As a final point, it must be remembered that compartment syndromes coexist with other injuries to the involved extremity. The treatment of the compartment syndrome is given top priority. The other injuries (e.g., fractures, dislocations, open wounds, burns), however, also must be managed according to the principles outlined in other chapters of this section.

33

ANKLE PAIN

C. Michael LeCroy

Pain in the ankle usually is associated with a history of specific antecedent trauma. Injuries to the ankle are common and range in severity from simple sprains to complex intraarticular fractures of the distal tibia. Along with knee trauma, ankle injuries commonly are encountered in recreational accidents. These injuries are the result of relatively low energy mechanisms of injury and generally carry a favorable prognosis. On the other hand, ankle trauma following high-energy mechanisms of injury can significantly impair extremity function. Like the knee and leg, the bone and soft tissue structures of the ankle are readily accessible for examination. Therefore accurate diagnosis usually is possible with careful physical examination.

■ PHONE CALL

Questions

1. **How was the ankle injured?**
   An understanding of the mechanism of injury is critical in the evaluation of musculoskeletal trauma. This is the initial step in the formulation of a differential diagnosis.
2. **Is there gross deformity?**
   Obvious deformity of the ankle usually indicates fracture or dislocation or both.
3. **Is there swelling?**
   Swelling apparent almost immediately after injury is a sign of significant bone or soft tissue trauma.
4. **Can the patient localize the pain?**
   The ability of the patient to localize the pain to a specific region can be very helpful in establishing a diagnosis. Not uncommonly, however, patients with ankle trauma will present with diffuse pain.
5. **Is there an associated skin wound or laceration?**
   An open wound should alert the physician to the potential for an open fracture or intraarticular communication, conditions that require urgent evaluation and treatment.
6. **Can the patient move the foot and toes of the injured leg?**
   Spontaneous or voluntary movement of the ipsilateral foot and toes distal to the site of injury can provide a rough assessment of whether there is concomitant neurologic injury. This must be evaluated subsequently by physical examination.

7. Is there a palpable distal pulse?

A palpable distal pulse can establish that blood flow is adequate distal to the site of injury. Although this does not rule out associated vascular trauma, it does signify sufficient peripheral circulation.

8. Can the patient ambulate on the injured leg?

A history of weight bearing on the injured leg makes a significant fracture or dislocation of the ankle highly unlikely.

9. Does the patient have any additional injuries?

As with all trauma to the musculoskeletal system, associated injuries to other body systems must be ruled out. This is particularly important in cases of high-energy trauma, in which the incidence of associated injuries is high.

10. Is the patient hemodynamically stable?

Hemodynamic stability is the first priority of management in all trauma victims. If the patient is not hemodynamically stable, attention should be turned to the ABCs (airway, breathing, circulation) before the musculoskeletal injury is evaluated.

Orders

1. Ask the RN to immobilize the ankle and lower leg, particularly if evaluation of the patient is going to be delayed for more than a few minutes. This will reduce pain and protect the extremity against further soft tissue injury. The ankle is most effectively immobilized with a posterior plaster splint. Rolled sheets or wooden splints also may be used, as may prefabricated splints. Care should be taken not to constrict the extremity with tight circumferential straps or bandages.

2. Ask the RN to elevate the injured ankle and foot above the level of the patient's heart. Elevation is critical in the treatment of ankle and foot injuries because of the tremendous potential for swelling and soft tissue compromise in these areas. The injured ankle should be elevated on pillows or sheets; alternatively, the foot of the bed can be elevated.

3. If the patient has sustained a high-energy mechanism of injury, such as a motor vehicle accident, ask the RN to obtain immediate consultation with a trauma specialist (emergency medicine physician or general surgeon).

Inform RN

"I will arrive at the bedside within 30 minutes."

Most ankle injuries are not limb threatening and generally do not require emergent evaluation. Urgent evaluation is indicated, however, if an open fracture or dislocation is suspected from the described injury mechanism and history. In general, to minimize

patient discomfort and optimize outcome, all ankle injuries should
be evaluated as soon as possible.

■ ELEVATOR THOUGHTS

Strains
- None

Sprains
- Lateral (inversion) ankle sprain
- Medial (eversion) ankle sprain

Dislocations
- Ankle (tibiotalar) dislocation

Fractures
- Ankle fractures
  Unimalleolar fracture (lateral or medial malleolus)
  Bimalleolar fracture (lateral and medial malleoli)
  Maisonneuve fracture (medial malleolus and proximal
     fibula)
  Trimalleolar fracture (lateral, medial, and posterior malleoli)
- Tibial plafond fracture (pilon fracture)

Other
- Achilles tendon rupture

■ BEDSIDE

Vital Signs

A complete set of vital signs is necessary in all trauma patients. In
general, an isolated injury to the ankle should not alter the vital
signs. As with trauma to other body regions, it should be expected
that pain and anxiety will elevate the blood pressure and heart rate.

Selective History

How was the ankle injured?
   Once the preliminary assessment is completed and hemodynamic stability assured, the examiner should attempt to obtain a
more detailed description of the mechanism of injury. Often an
understanding of how the injury occurred can lead to an
anatomic diagnosis. Ankle injuries are common following both
high- and low-energy mechanisms. Patients who describe a
twisting injury during recreational activities most often experience sprains. In contrast, high-energy mechanisms of trauma to
the ankle, such as motor vehicle crashes, can cause fracture or
dislocation. In twisting injuries to the ankle, an attempt should be

made to determine whether inversion or eversion forces were involved. With inversion injuries, lateral ligament injury or fracture should be suspected; conversely, with eversion injuries, medial injuries should be suspected. A history of direct axial force transmitted through the ankle during a motor vehicle accident should lead the physician to suspect a tibial plafond fracture. The Achilles tendon ruptures most often during recreational activity. If this injury is suspected, the patient should be asked whether any sound accompanied the trauma; many patients with heelcord ruptures note an audible "pop" at the time of injury.

What was the condition of the patient immediately following the injury?

It is helpful to determine the condition of the patient immediately after the injury. This information can be quite useful in establishing the potential for significant bone or soft tissue trauma to the ankle. For example, a history of weight bearing on the involved leg after the injury makes a significant fracture or dislocation highly unlikely. In contrast, a history of soft tissue swelling immediately after injury should elevate the examiner's suspicion for ligament disruption or fracture.

Can the patient localize the pain?

The patient should be asked to localize the pain if the site of injury is not immediately apparent (as with an open fracture or an obvious skeletal deformity). Many patients with ankle trauma will complain of diffuse pain and tenderness. Any ability of the patient to localize the point(s) of maximum discomfort, however, can assist in establishing the diagnosis. It is particularly helpful to determine whether the ankle is painful medially (eversion ankle injury), laterally (inversion ankle injury), or in both locations (bimalleolar injury). Similarly, pain localized to the posterior aspect of the ankle suggests Achilles tendon injury.

What are the patient-specific factors?

This final category of information is essential in the management of all patients with musculoskeletal trauma. The patient's age, occupation, past medical history, and functional demands should be determined. Any history of prior ankle injury must be identified so that the acute trauma can be distinguished from preexisting conditions. These factors considerably influence the prognosis as well as the treatment plan once the precise diagnosis is established.

Selective Physical Examination

Inspection

The patient may be examined while seated or while lying supine with both lower extremities exposed to above the knee. To begin the examination, it is helpful to briefly observe the patient from the foot of the bed to determine the degree of discomfort he or she is experiencing. This can assist the examiner in determining the potential for significant bone or soft tissue injury to the ankle. The physician should note any swelling, ecchymosis, or deformity, determining whether the ankle is swollen medially, laterally, or diffusely. With unstable ankle fractures and ankle dislocations, deformity usually is readily apparent. With sprains and stable fractures, however, the physical findings are more subtle. In evaluating the presence of deformity and swelling, it is often useful to compare the injured ankle to the contralateral uninjured one. The injured ankle should be inspected circumferentially for any loss of skin integrity. It must be ascertained whether any wounds or lacerations communicate with underlying fractures or articular surfaces. Finally, the patient should be observed for spontaneous movements of the ipsilateral foot and toes. Such movements usually indicate intact distal neurovascular status.

Palpation

The ankle should be palpated in a systematic fashion, and all areas of localized tenderness and swelling should be correlated with underlying anatomic structures. The contours of the lateral and medial malleoli should be palpated and notation made of tenderness medially, laterally, or in both locations. Because of the subcutaneous position of the malleoli, movement of fracture surfaces upon palpation can often be appreciated. The medial and lateral ligaments also should be palpated. Medially, the deltoid ligament courses from the medial malleolus to the medial hindfoot. Laterally, the two most important ligaments are the anterior talofibular ligament (anterior to the lateral malleolus) and the calcaneofibular ligament (posterior to the lateral malleolus). Significant swelling and tenderness over these ligaments suggests ligament injury.

The posterior aspect of the ankle should be palpated next. The Achilles tendon normally can be palpated as a thick band to its point of insertion onto the calcaneal tuberosity. In an Achilles tendon rupture, palpation reveals tenderness and a defect in the tendon. The Thompson calf squeeze test also should be performed in the evaluation of a possible Achilles tendon rupture (see Special Tests). Finally, in the evaluation of ankle injuries the examiner must remember to palpate the fibula along its entire course. This will assist in ruling out a high fibula fracture (Maisonneuve fracture) or an injury to the tibiofibular syndesmosis.

Movements

If ankle deformity is obvious, no attempt should be made to move the extremity. If, however, bone injury is not immediately apparent, the ankle joint should be moved gently through a range of dorsiflexion and plantar flexion. Significant pain with this maneuver or limitation of movement is a sign of musculoskeletal injury. Conversely, normal, pain-free range of motion usually rules out significant fracture or dislocation of the ankle. The ankle also should be tested with inversion and eversion stresses. Significant pain with inversion suggests a lateral injury, whereas pain with eversion indicates a medial injury. In complete ligament disruptions the examiner may appreciate total instability of the ankle either laterally (most common) or medially with inversion or eversion stresses.

If disruption of the Achilles tendon is suspected, active plantar flexion of the ankle also should be assessed. Inability to actively plantar flex corroborates heelcord disruption.

Special Tests

In addition to the basic principles of inspection, palpation, and assessment of movements, complete evaluation of the injured ankle requires several special maneuvers not applicable to other extremity injuries. It is important to emphasize that these tests should be performed on the uninjured ankle as well as the injured ankle, since this will allow for the appreciation of subtle differences and increase the sensitivity of the maneuvers.

Anterior Drawer Test.   This maneuver is designed to identify an injury to the anterior talofibular ligament. The test is performed by grasping the heel posteriorly and pulling anteriorly, thereby attempting to subluxate the talus from within the ankle mortise. An important point to remember is that the maneuver must be performed with the ankle in plantar flexion, thus relaxing the calcaneofibular ligament. Significant anterior displacement suggests complete anterior talofibular ligament disruption.

Thompson Test.   This test is the most sensitive physical finding in the diagnosis of complete rupture of the Achilles tendon. Ideally the Thompson test should be performed with the patient lying prone on the examining table and the ipsilateral knee flexed ninety degrees. The calf midportion is then squeezed firmly. If the heelcord is intact, this maneuver will elicit involuntary plantar flexion of the ankle. If the heelcord is disrupted, no plantar flexion will be observed.

Neurovascular Examination

A focused neurologic assessment of the injured extremity is necessary with ankle trauma to exclude concomitant neurologic injury. Injury to the peripheral nerves at the level of the ankle primarily will affect sensory function in the foot. Sensation should be tested in the distributions of the superficial peroneal, deep peroneal, and tibial nerves as described in Chapter 29.

Significant vascular injury is uncommon with ankle injuries. Even in the presence of an ankle dislocation with damage to the anterior tibial artery, adequate circulation to the foot normally is maintained via the posterior tibial artery and the collateral circulation. In patients with ankle trauma, significant soft tissue swelling may prevent direct palpation of the dorsalis pedis and posterior tibial pulses. If the pulses cannot be palpated, Doppler evaluation is indicated. As with all extremity injuries, capillary refill time in the digits of the involved extremity can verify the adequacy of distal circulation.

■ FURTHER ORDERS

All patients sustaining ankle trauma should be referred for radiographs. Standard screening radiographs of the ankle consist of AP, lateral, and mortise images. The mortise radiograph is an AP radiograph obtained with the ankle internally rotated 30 degrees. The importance of this view in the evaluation of ankle injuries cannot be overstated. The mortise image best illustrates the position of the talus within the ankle mortise and can demonstrate instability or subluxation not appreciable on other images. A Maisonneuve fracture suspected on the basis of physical examination may be definitively diagnosed with a supplemental AP radiograph of the ipsilateral knee that demonstrates the high fibula fracture.

If a complete disruption of the lateral ligaments is suspected (positive anterior drawer test), consideration should be given to obtaining an inversion stress radiograph of the ankle. This maneuver requires analgesia for the patient and should be performed either with general anesthesia (when applicable) or with an intraarticular injection of local anesthetic solution. The ankle is inverted maximally, and an AP radiograph is obtained. The contralateral uninjured ankle should be examined in the same manner (minus the anesthetic). Inversion of the talus 5 to 7 degrees more on the injured side than on the uninjured side is considered diagnostic of incompetence of the lateral ligament supports.

■ MANAGEMENT

Ankle injuries are common with high- and low-energy mechanisms. In general, high-energy mechanisms cause fractures or dislocations, whereas low-energy mechanisms cause soft tissue injuries (ligament damage). The focus of the initial evaluation of the patient with traumatic ankle pain should be to determine which of these types of injury the patient has sustained. Immediate orthopaedic consultation is indicated for all fractures of the ankle and tibial plafond and for dislocation of the ankle. On the other hand, ankle ligament injuries usually are managed most appropriately by a nonorthopaedist initially and by an orthopaedist for follow-up.

Ankle sprains are the most commonly encountered ankle injuries. An ankle sprain should be suspected in the patient with a history of a twisting mechanism of injury, swelling and tenderness on examination, and radiographs negative for fractures. Initial treatment of ligament injuries should be based on the amount of swelling and pain, with consideration given to patient-specific factors. Compressive bandages, plaster splints, prefabricated splints, and strapping are all used commonly to treat ankle sprains. All ankle sprains should be managed initially with compression (bandage or splint), elevation, and protected weight bearing. Cold therapy and NSAIDs may also be helpful acutely. If significant ligament disruption is suspected, such as a third-degree sprain, the patient should be placed into a posterior splint acutely followed later by a short-leg walking cast. Patients with severe ankle sprains should be referred for orthopaedic follow-up within 5 to 10 days. The focus of subsequent care is to regain ankle mobility and resume full weight bearing as soon as the pain and swelling have subsided. Acute surgical intervention is never indicated in the management of ankle sprains; late reconstruction, however, may be indicated for chronic ligament instability. Although the treatment of ankle sprains is relatively straightforward, the physician should remember that symptoms of ankle sprains can persist for months after the injury.

In the absence of ankle dislocation, the immediate management of ankle skeletal injury is immobilization of the extremity to minimize patient discomfort and prevent further soft tissue trauma. A plaster splint is the most effective means of immobilizing the ankle. A standard posterior splint consisting of splints along the plantar foot and posterior calf supplemented by a sugar tong splint across the ankle joint and extending along the medial and lateral aspects of the leg will effectively immobilize the ankle and maintain it in neutral position. Prefabricated splints also are available in many hospitals. All splints should be well padded to accommodate the anticipated soft tissue swelling.

Ankle dislocation should be considered an orthopaedic emergency (Fig. 33–1). These injuries can disrupt the blood supply to the dome of the talus. In addition, associated fractures of the ankle and talus are common. The tibiotalar joint should be reduced as soon as possible. Under ordinary circumstances this can be done in the emergency room with intravenous sedation or intraarticular injection of local anesthetic solution. These injuries should be considered unstable after reduction, even in the absence of associated fracture, and a plaster splint should be applied.

Ankle fractures are characterized by the extent of bone involvement and by whether there is associated ligament injury. The most appropriate treatment for fractures of the ankle is determined with consideration of the fracture pattern as well as the patient's bone quality and functional status. In general the recommended treatment is based on the amount of displacement of the talus within the ankle mortise and the perceived stability of the joint. Fractures involving lateral displacement of the talus within the mortise and bimalleolar fractures perceived to be unstable usually are managed with operative reduction and internal fixation. In contrast to the surgical treatment of many lower extremity fractures, surgical treatment of ankle fractures commonly is performed on a semi-elective basis.

Nonoperative management may be indicated for stable, nondisplaced ankle fractures and in patients not believed to be suitable surgical candidates. These patients commonly are managed with cast immobilization. If closed treatment is selected, care must be taken to avoid applying a circumferential cast to an acutely swollen extremity. Protected weight bearing is essential to the successful management of ankle fractures, regardless of whether treatment is operative or nonoperative.

Most ankle fractures involving either the lateral or medial malleolus—*unimalleolar fractures*—are stable and can be managed non-

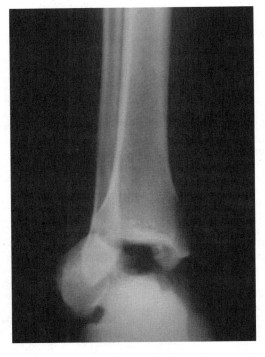

Figure 33–1 □ AP radiograph of the ankle illustrating complete tibiotalar (ankle) dislocation.

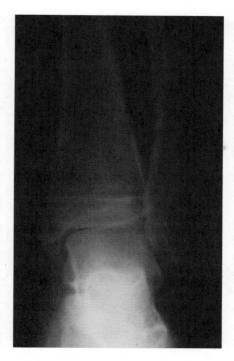

Figure 33–2 □ AP radiograph of the ankle demonstrating a bimalleolar fracture pattern with significant displacement of the ankle mortise.

operatively with cast immobilization if fracture displacement is minimal. Fractures involving both the lateral and medial malleoli—*bimalleolar fractures* (Fig. 33–2)—should be considered unstable even in the absence of fracture displacement, and operative stabilization is common. A fracture of the distal fibula with concomitant medial ligament injury—*a functional bimalleolar ankle fracture*—can lead to lateral subluxation of the talus and for this reason often requires operative fixation. *Trimalleolar ankle fractures,* involving the lateral, medial, and posterior malleoli, are managed best with operative reduction and internal fixation. Maisonneuve fractures exhibit tibiofibular syndesmotic disruption in addition to the medial malleolar fracture, and operative stabilization of the syndesmosis is often necessary.

Fractures involving the weight-bearing portion of the distal tibia (tibial plafond fractures) are among the most difficult injuries for orthopaedic surgeons to treat (Fig. 33–3). Characteristically these fractures are the result of high-energy trauma, exhibit bone com-

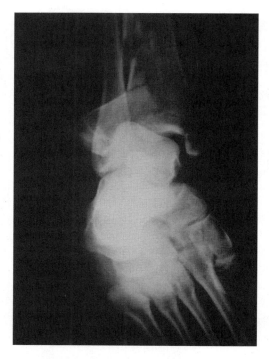

Figure 33–3 □ AP radiograph of the ankle illustrating a complex fracture of the distal tibial articular surface (tibial plafond fracture).

minution, and are associated with significant soft tissue injury. Operative treatment almost always is necessary, and long-term arthrosis and stiffness are common complications despite reduction and stabilization.

Emergent orthopaedic intervention is indicated for open fracture of the ankle or tibial plafond because of the high risk of infection. Open fractures require emergent operative debridement and appropriate skeletal stabilization. Any open wounds should be covered with a sterile povidone-iodine (Betadine)-soaked gauze dressing pending definitive operative management.

Rupture of the Achilles tendon may be managed effectively with either operative repair or closed treatment. Operative repair, which is elective, is associated with a lower incidence of rerupture, earlier return to activities, and greater plantar flexion strength. However, good results have also been obtained with nonoperative treatment of heelcord ruptures. Patients undergoing closed treatment are managed initially with an equinus cast (ankle in plantar flexion), followed by gradual return of the ankle to neutral position.

34

FOOT PAIN

C. Michael LeCroy

In contrast to complaints of pain in the leg and ankle, where trauma is the usual cause, pain in the foot most commonly arises from nontraumatic conditions. Foot pain, however, can also result from trauma to the lower extremity. High-energy mechanisms, such as falls, motor vehicle accidents, and crushing injuries, usually are implicated in these injuries. Foot pain following recreational trauma is relatively rare. Many of the wide variety of fractures and dislocations possible in the foot can be managed successfully with minimal intervention. Foot injuries are encountered frequently in association with other trauma to the musculoskeletal system. In these situations the foot injuries are often assigned a lower priority in the initial management of the multiply injured patient. Diligent and early intervention is indicated in all foot injuries, however, to prevent long-term complications.

In the evaluation of foot injuries the multitude of small bones and articulations makes anatomic diagnosis on the basis of physical examination alone challenging. By convention the foot is divided into three anatomic regions: the hindfoot, midfoot, and forefoot (Fig. 34–1). The junction between the hindfoot and midfoot is

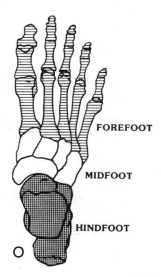

Figure 34–1 □ Anatomic regions of the foot. (From Weissman BNW, Sledge CB: Orthopedic Radiology. Philadelphia, WB Saunders, 1986, p 628.)

FOREFOOT

MIDFOOT

HINDFOOT

known as the transverse tarsal joint, or Chopart's joint. Similarly, the junction between the midfoot and forefoot is known as Lisfranc's joint. Each of these three regions of the foot has characteristic and widely varying patterns of injury.

■ PHONE CALL

Questions

1. **How was the foot injured?**

   An understanding of the mechanism of injury is critical in the evaluation of musculoskeletal trauma. This is the initial step in the formulation of a differential diagnosis.

2. **Is there gross deformity?**

   Obvious deformity of the foot usually indicates fracture or dislocation or both.

3. **Is there swelling?**

   Swelling apparent almost immediately after the injury is a sign of significant bone or soft tissue trauma.

4. **Can the patient localize the pain?**

   The ability of the patient to localize the pain to a specific region can be very helpful in establishing a diagnosis. Not uncommonly, however, patients with foot trauma present with diffuse pain.

5. **Is there an associated skin wound or laceration?**

   An open wound should alert the physician to the potential for an open fracture or intraarticular communication, conditions that require urgent evaluation and treatment because of the associated high risk of infection.

6. **Is there complete or near complete digital amputation?**

   These injuries should alert the physician to the likelihood of significant bone and soft tissue trauma to the foot. High-energy crushing and mangling mechanisms are normally responsible.

7. **Can the patient move the toes of the injured foot?**

   Spontaneous or voluntary movements of the toes distal to the site of injury can provide a rough assessment of whether there is concomitant neurovascular injury. The neurovascular status of the foot must be evaluated subsequently by physical examination.

8. **Is the dorsalis pedis pulse palpable?**

   A palpable dorsalis pedis pulse can establish that blood flow to the injured foot is adequate. Although this does not rule out associated vascular trauma, in most cases it does signify sufficient peripheral circulation.

9. **Was the patient ambulatory on the injured foot after the accident?**

   A history of weight bearing on the injured foot makes a

significant fracture or dislocation of the hindfoot unlikely. In contrast, ambulation may be possible with midfoot and fore-foot injuries.

10. Are there any associated injuries?

As with all trauma to the musculoskeletal system, associated injuries to the axial skeleton as well as to other body systems must be ruled out. This is particularly important for high-energy trauma to the foot, where the incidence of associated injuries is high.

11. Is the patient hemodynamically stable?

Hemodynamic stability is the first priority of management in all trauma victims. If the patient is not hemodynamically stable, attention should be turned to the ABCs (airway, breathing, circulation) before the musculoskeletal injury is evaluated.

Orders

1. Ask the RN to immobilize the foot and ankle, particularly if evaluation of the patient will be delayed for more than a few minutes. This will reduce pain and protect the foot against further soft tissue injury. The foot may be immobilized effectively with a posterior plaster splint or a prefabricated splint. Care should be taken not to constrict the foot with tight circumferential straps or bandages.

2. Ask the RN to elevate the injured foot and ankle above the level of the patient's heart. Elevation is critical in the treatment of foot injuries because of the tremendous potential for swelling and soft tissue compromise. The injured foot should be elevated on pillows or sheets; alternatively, the foot of the bed may be elevated. The only exception to the recommendation for elevation of the injured foot is suspected compartment syndrome, as discussed in Chapter 32.

3. If the patient has sustained a high-energy mechanism of injury, as in a motor vehicle accident or a fall from a height, ask the RN to obtain immediate consultation with a trauma specialist (emergency medicine physician or general surgeon).

Inform RN

"I will arrive at the bedside within 30 minutes."

Most foot injuries are not limb threatening and generally do not require urgent evaluation. If an open fracture is suspected from the described injury mechanism and history, however, urgent evaluation is indicated. Also, suspected compartment syndrome in the foot following crush injury must be evaluated and treated urgently to prevent irreversible muscle necrosis and compromised limb function. In general, to minimize patient discomfort and optimize outcome, all foot injuries should be evaluated as soon as possible.

■ ELEVATOR THOUGHTS

Strains
- None

Sprains
- Midfoot sprain (tarsometatarsal joints)
- Forefoot sprain (metatarsophalangeal joints)
- Phalangeal sprain (jammed toe, interphalangeal joints)

Dislocations
- Hindfoot
    Subtalar dislocation (talocalcaneal joint)
- Midfoot
    Chopart's dislocations
        Talonavicular dislocation
        Calcaneocuboid dislocation
    Lisfranc's dislocations (tarsometatarsal joints)
- Forefoot
    Metatarsophalangeal dislocation
    Interphalangeal dislocation

Fractures
- Hindfoot
    Talar body fracture
    Talar neck fracture
    Calcaneal fracture
- Midfoot
    Navicular fracture
    Cuboid fracture
    Cuneiform fracture
- Forefoot
    Metatarsal fracture
    Phalangeal fracture

Other
- Compartment syndrome of foot
- Amputation or near amputation of digit

■ BEDSIDE

Vital Signs

A complete set of vital signs is necessary in any trauma patient. In general, an isolated injury to the foot should not alter the vital signs. As with trauma to other body regions, it should be anticipated that pain and anxiety will elevate the blood pressure and heart rate.

Selective History

How exactly was the foot injured?
Once the preliminary assessment has been completed and hemodynamic stability assured, the examiner should attempt to obtain a more detailed description of the mechanism of injury. Often an understanding of how the injury occurred can lead to an anatomic diagnosis. Most foot injuries are the result of high-energy mechanisms such as falls, motor vehicle crashes, crushing injuries, or mangling lacerations (e.g., lawnmower injuries). In a fall from a significant height a tremendous force may be transmitted through the hindfoot. Fractures of the calcaneus are common in this setting. Talar neck fractures and Lisfranc's fracture-dislocations are the most common foot injuries noted following high-speed motor vehicle crashes when the foot is braced against the floorboard at the time of impact. Crushing injuries to the foot characteristically inflict significant soft tissue as well as bone trauma. Multiple metatarsal fractures are common with crush injuries, which also carry a high risk of compartment syndrome. Mangling injuries to the foot usually involve trauma to one or more phalanges. If the patient with posttraumatic foot pain presents without a definite history of high-energy trauma, such as the mechanisms described above, isolated phalangeal fractures or sprains should be suspected.

What was the condition of the patient immediately following the injury?
The condition of the patient following the injury can help establish the potential for significant bone or soft tissue trauma to the foot. For example, a history of full weight bearing on the injured foot makes the diagnosis of a dislocation or fracture of the hindfoot or midfoot unlikely. In contrast, a history of soft tissue swelling immediately after the injury and inability to bear weight suggest significant fracture or dislocation.

Can the patient localize the pain?
The patient should be asked to localize the pain if the site of injury is not immediately apparent (as with an open fracture or an obvious skeletal deformity). Many patients with foot trauma complain of diffuse pain and tenderness. If the patient can localize the point(s) of maximum discomfort, however, it will assist in establishing the diagnosis. Pain localized to the heel may indicate calcaneal fracture. Symptoms localized to the ball of the foot suggest a Lisfranc injury. Pain along the lateral aspect of the midfoot may indicate a fracture of the fifth metatarsal base.

What are the patient-specific factors?
This category of information is essential in the management of all patients with musculoskeletal trauma. The patient's age, oc-

cupation, past medical history, and functional demands should be determined. A history of diabetes mellitus increases the potential for infection and raises the possibility of neuropathic (Charcot's) fractures. A history of cigarette smoking increases the risk of complications of bone and soft tissue healing. Any history of prior foot injury also must be identified so that acute trauma can be distinguished from preexisting conditions. Although these patient-specific factors usually will not establish the diagnosis, they are quite useful in formulating a treatment plan and prognosis once the diagnosis has been made.

Selective Physical Examination

Inspection

The patient may be examined while seated or lying supine with both lower extremities exposed to above the knee. Observing the patient briefly from the foot of the bed can help determine the degree of discomfort the patient is experiencing and thus the potential for significant bone or ligament injury to the foot. Any swelling, ecchymosis, or deformity should be noted. In fractures and dislocations of the hindfoot, deformity usually is readily apparent. In many foot injuries, however, the physical findings are more subtle. In evaluating deformity and swelling, it is often useful to compare the injured foot to the contralateral uninjured one. The injured foot should be inspected circumferentially to rule out any loss of skin integrity on either the dorsal or plantar surfaces. It must be ascertained whether any wounds or lacerations communicate with underlying fracture or articular surfaces. Finally the foot should be observed for spontaneous movements of the ipsilateral toes. Such movements usually indicate intact distal neurovascular status.

Palpation

The foot should be palpated in a systematic fashion, beginning with the hindfoot and proceeding distally to the midfoot and forefoot. An attempt should be made to palpate the major bones and articulations. All areas of localized tenderness and swelling should be correlated with underlying anatomic structures. Because of the subcutaneous position of many bones of the foot, movement of fracture surfaces on palpation often can be appreciated. The examiner also should palpate the foot circumferentially and determine the degree of swelling of the various muscle compartments. Significant circumferential swelling and pain with palpation should raise the index of suspicion for compartment syndrome of the foot.

Movements

If there is obvious deformity of the foot, no attempt should be made to move the extremity. If, however, skeletal injury is not immediately apparent, the foot and ankle should be moved gently through a range of dorsiflexion and plantar flexion of the hindfoot, midfoot, and forefoot sequentially. Significant pain with these maneuvers or limitation of movement is a sign of musculoskeletal injury. In contrast, full and pain-free range of motion usually rules out significant fracture or dislocation of the foot. If compartment syndrome of the foot is suspected on the basis of the injury mechanism and physical findings, the patient should be evaluated for pain with passive stretch. This may be accomplished by stabilizing the hindfoot and passively flexing and extending the toes. Significant pain with this maneuver is the most sensitive physical finding in the diagnosis of compartment syndrome, as discussed in Chapter 32.

Neurovascular Examination

A focused neurovascular assessment of the injured extremity is necessary with foot trauma to exclude concomitant neurovascular injury. Injury to the peripheral nerves at the level of the foot will affect only sensory function. Sensation should be tested in the distributions of the superficial peroneal, deep peroneal, and tibial nerves as described in Chapter 29. In addition, sensation should be assessed in the distributions of the saphenous nerve (medial hindfoot) and sural nerve (lateral hindfoot). Significant vascular injury is uncommon with injuries to the foot, primarily because of the abundant collateral circulation. The posterior tibial artery may be injured with subtalar dislocation, but adequate peripheral circulation is maintained via the dorsalis pedis artery. In trauma to the foot, significant soft tissue swelling may prevent direct palpation of the dorsalis pedis and posterior tibial pulses. If the pulses cannot be palpated, Doppler evaluation is indicated. Capillary refill time may also be assessed in the digits of the injured foot to ensure the adequacy of distal circulation.

General Physical Examination

Injuries to more than one region of the musculoskeletal system are common following high-energy trauma. For this reason a thorough examination of the entire musculoskeletal system is necessary in the evaluation of extremity trauma. This is particularly relevant in the evaluation of foot trauma. The importance of carefully examining the patient with foot trauma for other skeletal injuries cannot be overstated. Consideration should be given especially to the potential for concomitant spine injury, pelvic ring disruption, and lower extremity long bone fractures.

■ FURTHER ORDERS

All foot injuries require referral for radiographs. Standard screening radiographs of the foot consist of AP, lateral, and oblique images. Most foot fractures and dislocations can be identified adequately and characterized on these three images. If calcaneal fracture is identified, an axial radiograph of the heel should be obtained also to further characterize the fracture pattern and displacement. Further radiographic studies, such as a CT scan, may be indicated in the evaluation of certain foot injuries, particularly intraarticular calcaneal fractures and talar neck fractures. In general the decision to obtain such studies should be made after consultation with the treating orthopaedic surgeon.

■ MANAGEMENT

The initial focus in the evaluation of the patient with a foot injury, as with other extremity trauma, is to determine whether there is a fracture or dislocation. A foot sprain should be suspected in the patient with a history of foot injury, swelling and tenderness on examination, and radiographs negative for fracture or dislocation. In general, sprains of the foot are managed best symptomatically with light compression, cold therapy, elevation, and NSAIDs. A brief period of protected weight bearing with crutches may also be indicated based on the amount of discomfort the patient is experiencing. Patients should be instructed to resume full weight bearing as soon as their symptoms allow. Long-term immobilization of the foot rarely is indicated in the management of soft tissue trauma. Physical therapy may help the patient resume weight bearing and regain range of motion of the foot.

One important point regarding foot sprains is that the physician should not be cavalier in the management of a midfoot sprain. Patients with foot trauma and symptoms of tenderness and swelling in the region of the tarsometatarsal joints should be considered at high risk for a Lisfranc injury. The radiographic findings in these injuries may be subtle, and orthopaedic consultation should be obtained if a Lisfranc fracture-dislocation cannot be definitively excluded. As discussed below, Lisfranc injuries usually require operative treatment.

A dislocation of the hindfoot or midfoot should be considered an orthopaedic emergency, and immediate consultation is indicated. Subtalar dislocations may be either medial or lateral and often are associated with open wounds and fractures of the hindfoot. In addition, these injuries can disrupt the blood supply to the dome of the talus, leading to osteonecrosis. The subtalar joint dislocation should be reduced as soon as possible. If there are associated open wounds or fractures and if the operating room is available, the dislocation should be reduced using general anesthesia in the operating room. If an operating room is not available, the dislocation can be reduced in the emergency department using intravenous sedation and local anesthesia. The physician should be prepared, however, for the possibility that a closed reduction may not be possible because of interposed soft tissues either medially or laterally. Following reduction, all subtalar dislocations should be immobilized with either a plaster splint or, in unstable cases, an external fixator.

Dislocations of the transverse tarsal joints (Chopart's dislocations) are relatively uncommon. When seen, these injuries invariably are associated with high-energy trauma and multiple fractures and dislocations in the foot. The talonavicular and calcaneocuboid articulations should be reduced as soon as possible. Under normal circumstances this can be accomplished using closed techniques. If intraarticular fractures are also present, the reduction may be unstable and operative intervention may be necessary.

Dislocations and fracture-dislocations of the tarsometatarsal joints are known as Lisfranc injuries (Fig. 34–2). These injuries, if not recognized and treated appropriately, frequently are associated with long-term complications of midfoot pain and stiffness. The radiographic findings in these injuries may be subtle, and the diag-

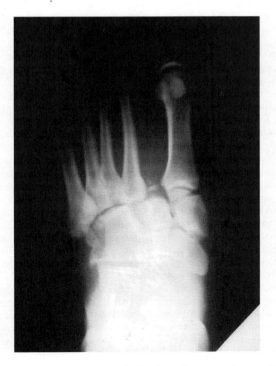

Figure 34–2 □ AP radiograph of the foot demonstrating multiple tarsometatarsal joint (Lisfranc) dislocations.

nosis can be missed. When recognized, Lisfranc injuries require operative intervention for reduction and stabilization of the tarsometatarsal articulations. This usually is accomplished with a combination of open and closed techniques.

Dislocations in the region of the forefoot (metatarsophalangeal and interphalangeal articulations) rarely require surgical intervention. These dislocations are successfully reduced in the emergency department with only local anesthesia (intraarticular local anesthetic injection or digital block). The joints are usually stable following reduction. Patients should be treated after reduction with light compression, elevation, NSAIDs, and orthopaedic follow-up in 5 to 7 days.

Fractures of the foot should be managed in the same manner as dislocations. Immediate orthopaedic consultation is indicated for fractures involving the hindfoot or midfoot. On the other hand, forefoot fractures often can be managed initially by a nonorthopaedist with referral for orthopaedic follow-up. Nonoperative management usually includes a posterior splint, elevation, and protected weight bearing. As with all foot injuries, physical therapy may be helpful in the rehabilitation phase to assist the patient with return to full weight bearing and to help restore range of motion.

Fractures of the talar neck are the result of high-energy forces. These injuries may be associated with disruptions of the subtalar, tibiotalar, and talonavicular articulations. Displaced talar neck fractures (Fig. 34–3) also frequently result in osteonecrosis of the talar dome because of disruption of the talar blood supply at the time of injury. Nondisplaced fractures of the talar neck may be treated nonoperatively, usually with a period of cast immobilization and non-weight-bearing status. Displaced talar neck fractures, in contrast, require urgent operative reduction and stabilization to minimize the risk of osteonecrosis and posttraumatic arthrosis. Fractures of the talar body are much less common. These injuries are not associated with disruption of talar vascularity and most often can be managed nonoperatively.

Fractures of the calcaneus (Fig. 34–4) present a unique challenge to the orthopaedist. These injuries, which are caused by high-energy forces, can be the source of lifelong pain and disability. Most extraarticular calcaneal fractures are managed best nonoperatively with a brief period of splinting followed by early range of motion exercises. There is considerable controversy among orthopaedists regarding the optimum treatment of intraarticular calcaneal fractures. These injuries traditionally have been treated with brief immobilization, protected weight bearing, and early range of motion exercises. In recent years, however, numerous authors have recommended open reduction and internal fixation in the management of these fractures. The advantages of operative vs. nonoperative treatment are currently being investigated and debated. As

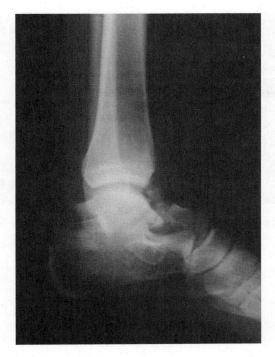

Figure 34–3 □ Lateral radiographs of the ankle and hindfoot with a displaced fracture of the talar neck.

with all musculoskeletal injuries, patient-specific factors play a significant role in the decision whether to operate. Operative treatment usually is performed 5 or more days after the injury, after the acute swelling has subsided. Patients are managed in the interim with a bulky, compressive cotton wrap, a posterior splint, strict elevation, and non-weight-bearing status.

Fractures of the midfoot are much less common than fractures of the hindfoot and are associated with less long-term disability. Most of these fractures are managed effectively with a splint or cast, elevation, NSAIDs, and progression to full weight bearing once the acute symptoms have subsided. Operative intervention occasionally may be indicated in the management of fractures of the navicular and cuboid to maintain the lengths of the medial and lateral columns of the foot, respectively.

Forefoot fractures (metatarsal and phalangeal fractures) usually are managed nonoperatively, and initial treatment by a non-orthopaedist is appropriate. Care must be taken to ensure that fractures at the bases of the metatarsals do not represent a Lisfranc in-

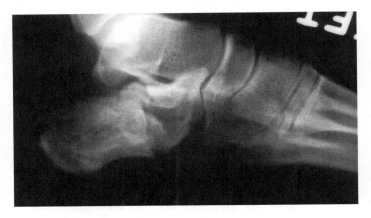

Figure 34–4 □ Lateral radiograph of the ankle and hindfoot illustrating an intraarticular fracture of the calcaneus.

jury. The conservative management of forefoot fractures consists of application of a posterior splint, followed by early conversion to a wooden-soled healing shoe. Elevation and NSAIDs are important in the management of these injuries, and weight bearing is encouraged as soon as symptoms allow. Fractures of the fifth metatarsal base are among the most commonly encountered forefoot fractures. These injuries may be avulsion fractures at the insertion of the peroneus brevis tendon or fractures at the proximal metaphyseal-diaphyseal junction. The avulsion fracture may be treated as described for other forefoot fractures. The fracture at the metaphyseal-diaphyseal junction, however, known as a Jones fracture, has a high incidence of nonunion and requires prolonged cast immobilization and protected weight bearing. Operative intervention occasionally may be indicated in cases of multiple metatarsal fractures and fractures of the first and fifth metatarsal shafts with loss of length of the medial or lateral columns of the foot or of both.

Open fracture of the foot requires emergent orthopaedic consultation because of the associated high risk of infection. Patients with open hindfoot or midfoot fractures require emergent operative debridement in addition to skeletal stabilization. Open fractures of the forefoot that would not otherwise require operative intervention may be managed in the emergency department with irrigation and debridement, depending on the judgment of the treating orthopaedist. Any open wounds should be covered with a sterile povidone-iodine (Betadine)-soaked gauze dressing pending definitive management.

Amputation or near amputation of toes may result from mangling injuries to the foot. These injuries should be managed with operative debridement to remove all devitalized bone and soft tissue, thereby reducing the risk of infection. Rarely is replantation of an amputated toe indicated. Amputation of a toe is not analogous to amputation of a finger, since excellent function may be realized with loss of one or more toes.

Finally, if compartment syndrome of the foot is suspected on the basis of the mechanism of injury and the physical examination findings, emergent orthopaedic consultation is necessary. A compartment syndrome must be treated with emergent fasciotomy. Compartment syndromes are discussed in more detail in Chapter 32.

35

NUMBNESS IN THE LEGS AND FEET

C. Michael LeCroy

Loss of sensation below the knee may follow injury to the back, pelvis, or legs. A variety of factors could be responsible, representing injury at different levels of the neurologic system from the spinal cord to the peripheral nerves. A thorough physical examination, combined with a detailed neurologic assessment of the lower extremities, is necessary to establish the correct diagnosis. The first priority of the examiner is to determine whether there actually is a neurologic deficit. Not uncommonly, patients with lower extremity trauma will describe vague subjective symptoms of numbness due to swelling in the extremity, pain, and apprehension. If the patient is discovered to have diminished sensation, the examiner's next priority is to determine the anatomic distribution of the sensory disturbance and to ascertain whether there are associated motor deficits. Numbness in the absence of paresis usually indicates minor neurologic injury with a good functional outcome expected. On the other hand, numbness combined with a motor deficit indicates more significant neurologic injury from which recovery is less certain.

■ PHONE CALL

Questions

1. **How did the injury occur?**
   An understanding of the mechanism of injury is critical in the evaluation of musculoskeletal trauma. This is the initial step in the formulation of a differential diagnosis.
2. **What is the pattern of the numbness?**
   A determination must be made of whether the patient is experiencing numbness in one or both legs and whether the diminished sensation involves the entire leg or an isolated portion (e.g., toes, foot, calf, thigh). This information is essential in establishing the level of neurologic injury.
3. **Do the symptoms follow a radicular pattern?**
   Radicular-like symptoms of radiating pain and intermittent tingling can be signs of nerve root involvement within the spinal canal.
4. **Can the patient move the foot and toes of the affected leg?**
   Spontaneous or voluntary movements of the foot and toes of the involved extremity(ies) can provide a rough assessment of whether there are concomitant motor deficits. This

must be evaluated subsequently by thorough physical examination.

5. Is the patient also complaining of pain in the back, pelvis, or lower extremities?

Complaints of localized pain can be helpful in determining what musculoskeletal injury may be responsible for the diminished sensation.

6. Is there gross deformity?

Obvious deformity of the spine, pelvis, or lower extremities usually indicates fracture or dislocation or both, injuries that may be responsible for the disturbance in lower extremity sensation.

7. Is there an associated skin wound or laceration?

An open lower extremity wound should alert the physician to the potential for direct peripheral nerve injury. In addition, such wounds may indicate an open fracture.

8. Does the patient have any additional injuries?

As with all trauma to the musculoskeletal system, associated injuries to other body systems must be excluded. This is particularly important in cases of high-energy trauma, in which the incidence of associated injuries is high.

9. Is the patient hemodynamically stable?

Hemodynamic stability is the first priority of management in all trauma victims. The potential for hemodynamic instability is particularly great in patients with spine, pelvis, or major lower extremity injuries. If the patient is not hemodynamically stable, attention should be turned to the ABCs (airway, breathing, circulation) before the musculoskeletal injury is evaluated.

Orders

1. If a spine injury is suspected from the mechanism of injury, the back should be immobilized by placing the patient supine on a rigid spine board. When placing or removing a spine board, assistance is necessary, and care must be taken to logroll the patient so that the entire spine and torso move as a single unit.

2. If obvious swelling or deformity is noted in the lower extremity(ies), ask the RN to immobilize the area of injury with plaster or prefabricated splints. The injured lower extremity should also be elevated.

3. If a skin laceration is noted on one or both lower extremities, ask the RN to apply a sterile compressive dressing.

4. If the patient has sustained a high-energy mechanism of injury, such as a motor vehicle accident, ask the RN to obtain immediate consultation with a trauma specialist (emergency medicine physician or general surgeon).

Inform RN

"I will arrive at the bedside immediately."

Complaints of numbness in the lower extremities following injury, whether due to swelling and apprehension or to an actual neurologic lesion, indicate significant injury to the musculoskeletal system. These symptoms may herald unstable injuries to the thoracolumbar spine or pelvis—injuries that may themselves be life threatening or associated with significant morbidity. For this reason, all patients with complaints of diminished lower extremity sensation should be evaluated on an urgent basis.

■ ELEVATOR THOUGHTS

- Pain or apprehension
    - Patients with fractures or dislocations of the lower extremity may describe subjective symptoms of numbness despite intact neurologic function
- Dislocations: *Neurologic injury in association with major joint dislocation*
    - Sacroiliac joint diastasis or disruption (L5 nerve root injury)
    - Hip dislocation (sciatic nerve injury)
    - Knee dislocation (tibial or common peroneal nerve injury)
    - Ankle dislocation (tibial, superficial peroneal, or deep peroneal nerve injury)
- Fractures: *Neurologic injury in association with pelvic ring or lower extremity fracture*
    - Sacral fracture (L4, L5, or S1 nerve root injury)
    - Acetabular fracture (sciatic nerve injury)
    - Distal femur fracture (tibial or common peroneal nerve injury)
    - Tibial shaft fracture (tibial nerve injury)
    - Fibular neck fracture (common peroneal nerve injury)
- High neurologic injuries
    - Thoracic spine injury (spinal cord injury)
    - Lumbosacral spine injury (involvement of L4, L5, S1 nerve roots)
    - Cauda equina syndrome
    - Lumbosacral plexus injury
- Isolated peripheral nerve injuries (*Any peripheral nerve may be injured by a direct blow, laceration, or projectile*)
    - Tibial nerve injury
    - Superficial peroneal nerve injury
    - Deep peroneal nerve injury
    - Sural nerve injury
    - Saphenous nerve injury
- Other
    - Compartment syndrome of thigh
    - Compartment syndrome of leg

■ BEDSIDE

Vital Signs

A complete set of vital signs is necessary in all trauma patients. It must be remembered that complaints of diminished lower extremity sensation can indicate significant musculoskeletal injury with the potential for hemodynamic instability. As with trauma to all body regions, it should be expected that pain and anxiety will elevate the blood pressure and heart rate.

Selective History

How exactly did the injury occur?

Once the preliminary assessment is completed and hemodynamic stability of the patient has been assured, the examiner should attempt to elicit as much information as possible regarding the mechanism of injury. This information can be helpful in narrowing the differential diagnosis in the patient with posttraumatic lower extremity numbness. For example, a patient with one or more lacerations to the lower extremity(ies) may have sustained direct injury to one or more peripheral nerves. On the other hand, a victim of a high-speed motor vehicle crash without lower extremity lacerations may have sustained a lumbosacral spine injury or pelvic ring disruption with an associated neurologic lesion. Any high-energy trauma to the lower extremities may cause a fracture or dislocation that injures a peripheral nerve. A patient who has sustained significant blunt trauma to the thigh or leg and who complains of lower extremity numbness should be considered at high risk for a compartment syndrome.

What is the pattern of numbness in the lower extremity(ies)?

The patient should be questioned carefully and asked to characterize the pattern of lower extremity sensory disturbance. If both legs are involved, a peripheral nerve or lumbosacral plexus injury is unlikely and the examiner should suspect trauma at the level of the lumbosacral spine. If only one lower extremity is involved, the physician should attempt to identify the portion of the leg or foot involved. This information can be helpful in differentiating between nerve root and peripheral nerve injuries. Particular attention should be paid to complaints of numbness in a nonanatomic distribution (e.g., entire leg below knee), as such complaints may indicate fictitious neurologic deficit. Finally the patient should also be questioned regarding radiating pain and tingling or numbness (paresthesias). Such symptoms usually indicate proximal neurologic injury at the nerve root level.

Can the patient localize any associated pain?

Most patients with posttraumatic lower extremity numbness also will complain of pain in the back, pelvis, or lower extremities. The patient should be asked to localize the pain as much as possible if the site of injury is not immediately apparent (as with open wounds or obvious skeletal deformity). The ability of the patient to localize pain can be helpful in determining the musculoskeletal injury responsible for the neurologic deficit. Pain localized to the back or pelvis points to a proximal neurologic injury as the source of the lower extremity numbness. On the other hand, symptoms localized to the long bones or joints may implicate an extremity fracture or dislocation as the cause.

What are the patient-specific factors?

As with all musculoskeletal trauma, knowledge of factors specific to the individual patient is vital. The patient's age, occupation, past medical history, and functional demands should be determined. Particular attention should be paid to any previous history of back pain, sciatica, herniated disc, or lower extremity trauma. Identification of these conditions can help distinguish acute trauma from preexisting conditions and may explain the lower extremity sensory disturbance. Even if this patient-specific information does not establish the diagnosis, it will be helpful in formulating a plan of treatment and prognosis once the diagnosis has been determined.

Selective Physical Examination

Inspection

The patient should be lying supine on the stretcher or spine board. All clothing should be removed to allow complete exposure of the back, pelvis, and lower extremities. Much useful information, including the degree of discomfort the patient is experiencing, can be gained by simply observing the patient from the foot of the bed for a few seconds. Most patients with a major fracture or dislocation of the spine, pelvis, or lower extremities will exhibit significant discomfort. The patient should be carefully observed also for spontaneous movements of the lower extremities. This can prove helpful in determining the presence and extent of motor deficits. Any swelling, ecchymosis, or deformity should be noted, as well as the location of any lacerations. If the lower extremity trauma is isolated, it is useful to compare the injured extremity to the contralateral uninjured one. All this information can assist in the identification of the musculoskeletal injury responsible for the alteration of lower extremity sensibility.

Palpation

The back, pelvis, and both lower extremities should be palpated systematically, beginning centrally at the spine and proceeding peripherally to the distal aspect of the lower extremities. If the patient is on a spine board because of suspected or potential spine trauma, the patient should be carefully logrolled to allow visual inspection and palpation of the thoracic and lumbosacral spine. Criteria for removal of the spine board should be followed (see Chapter 27). During palpation of the back, pelvis, and lower extremities, an attempt should be made to correlate all areas of localized swelling and tenderness with underlying anatomic structures. In the lower extremities, movement of fractured bone surfaces may be appreciated with gentle palpation. If compartment syndrome of the thigh or leg is considered a possibility because of the mechanism of injury, particular attention should be paid to palpation of the respective muscle compartments. Diffuse and marked swelling with tenderness may indicate a developing compartment syndrome. Finally, in the patient with suspected spine or pelvic trauma, a systematic examination with palpation from head to toe is indicated because of the high incidence of associated injuries in these patients.

Movements

In the evaluation of the patient with posttraumatic numbness of the leg, movement should be assessed in both lower extremities. In the absence of obvious deformity, the hip, knee, and ankle joints should be taken through a passive range of motion. Significant pain or limitation of motion with any of these maneuvers may help identify the injury responsible for the diminished sensation and will serve to focus the subsequent radiographic examination. Patients with no pain and full range of motion of all joints of the lower extremities can be assumed to have no fracture or dislocation. If compartment syndrome of the thigh or leg is suspected to be the source of the diminished sensation, the distal lower extremities should be evaluated for pain with passive stretch, which is the most sensitive test for compartment syndrome. The evaluation of active movements of the lower extremities is discussed in the following section.

Neurologic Examination

A thorough neurologic examination is the crux of the evaluation of the patient with posttraumatic lower extremity numbness. A complete understanding of the anatomy and patterns of innervation in the lower extremities is essential. It must be remembered that sensation in the leg and foot is under the control of the L4, L5, and S1 nerve roots centrally and the tibial, superficial peroneal, deep peroneal, sural, and saphenous nerves peripherally (Fig. 35–1).

The first priority of the neurologic examination is to determine whether there is a sensory deficit. Occasionally, patients who have sustained injury to the lower extremities or axial skeleton will describe vague symptoms of numbness in a nonanatomic distribution. These patients must be distinguished from those with an actual neurologic deficit. Sensation to both pin prick and light touch

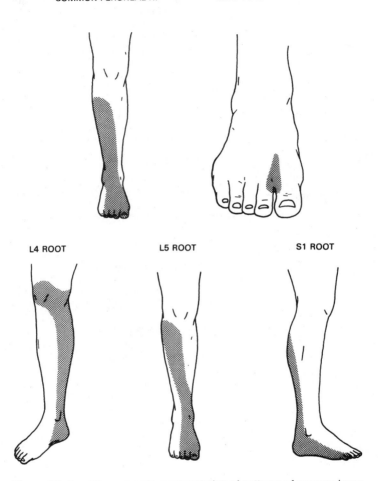

Figure 35–1 □ Diagrammatic representation of patterns of sensory innervation in the lower extremity. (From Birnbaum JS: The Musculoskeletal Manual, 2nd ed. Philadelphia, WB Saunders, 1986, pp 152–153.)

should be tested systematically in the leg and foot. All nerve root and peripheral nerve distributions should be assessed. A useful technique is to reserve testing of the portion of the leg or foot that the patient describes as "numb" for last and first evaluate sensation in the uninvolved portion of the lower extremity. The anatomic distribution of the diminished sensation should be noted. Comparison should be made to sensation in the contralateral lower extremity when appropriate.

Once a sensory disturbance has been confirmed and its anatomic distribution characterized, the next priority of the neurologic examination is to determine if there are concomitant motor deficits. Motor function should be assessed in both legs and feet with respect to the L4, L5, and S1 nerve roots, as well as to the tibial, superficial peroneal, and deep peroneal nerves. Motor function should be graded using the standard scheme (see Table 21–1).

The following list briefly summarizes the major sensory and motor functions of the nerve roots and peripheral nerves below the knee. These quick screening tests are useful in the characterization of neurologic deficit in the lower extremities. It should be remembered that neurologic deficit in both lower extremities usually indicates a high neurologic injury at the level of the spinal cord or cauda equina.

Nerve Roots
- **L4 Nerve root**
   Sensory: medial aspect of lower leg
   Motor: dorsiflexion of ankle
- **L5 Nerve root**
   Sensory: lateral aspect of lower leg, dorsum of foot
   Motor: dorsiflexion of great toe
- **S1 Nerve root**
   Sensory: sole of foot
   Motor: plantar flexion of ankle

Peripheral Nerves
- **Tibial nerve**
   Sensory: sole of foot (medial and lateral plantar nerves)
   Motor: plantar flexion of ankle (gastrocnemius-soleus complex)
- **Superficial peroneal nerve**
   Sensory: dorsum of foot
   Motor: ankle eversion (peroneal muscles)
- **Deep peroneal nerve**
   Sensory: first webspace dorsum of foot
   Motor: great toe extension (extensor hallucis longus)
- **Sural nerve**
   Sensory: lateral aspect of hindfoot
   Motor: none
- **Saphenous nerve**
   Sensory: medial aspect of hindfoot
   Motor: none

■ FURTHER ORDERS

No standard radiographs are indicated in the evaluation of the patient with posttraumatic numbness in the leg and foot. Rather, the need for radiographs is determined by the history and physical examination of the individual patient. Such radiographs often will reveal the skeletal injury responsible for the neurologic deficit. If fracture or dislocation of the spine, pelvis, or lower extremities is suspected, routine screening radiographs should be obtained of the suspected injury area as detailed in preceding chapters.

■ MANAGEMENT

The immediate management of the patient with posttraumatic numbness in the legs and feet involves determining whether there actually is a neurologic deficit and if so its pattern. Patients without true sensory deficits should be managed with analgesic medications and primary attention to any other injuries. On the other hand, if the patient is determined to have true neurologic deficit, immediate orthopaedic consultation is indicated. The focus of the subsequent management then becomes the identification and treatment of associated musculoskeletal injuries. Acute intervention for the neurologic injury itself rarely is indicated.

Concomitant motor deficits significantly affect the prognosis of posttraumatic lower extremity numbness. Many patients will present initially with complaints of numbness or tingling in the foot but no associated motor weakness. These patients can be assumed to have a neurapraxia rather than a complete nerve injury, and the prognosis for recovery of sensation is good with expectant treatment. On the other hand, when the patient is found to have motor weakness in association with complaints of numbness, the prognosis is less certain. Such patients likely have sustained a significant stretch or compressive injury to neurologic structures, and a prolonged course with slow and potentially incomplete recovery of neurologic function should be anticipated. In general, the prognosis is worse for these types of neurologic injuries in the lower extremity than in the upper extremity. Although acute intervention seldom is indicated for neurologic injuries with sensory and motor involvement, electrical studies (electromyography, nerve conduction studies) often are performed on a delayed basis to evaluate the severity of neurologic injury and the potential for recovery.

If the patient is found to have a neurologic deficit involving both lower extremities, a proximal neurologic injury at the level of the spinal cord or cauda equina should be suspected. The patient must be evaluated carefully for concomitant thoracic or lumbosacral spine injury as well as for traumatic intervertebral disk herniation. The principles and techniques of management of these injuries are discussed in Chapter 27.

Cauda equina syndrome is due to compression of the nerve roots in the spinal canal below the level of the spinal cord. This syndrome is characterized by bowel or bladder dysfunction (usually urinary retention), saddle anesthesia, and varying degrees of loss of lower extremity motor and sensory function. Cauda equina syndrome most commonly is caused by nontraumatic lumbar disk herniation; however, it can be due to lumbosacral spine trauma. Once a diagnosis of cauda equina syndrome has been made, emergent surgical decompression is necessary to arrest progression of neurologic deficit.

Disruptions of the pelvic ring also can be associated with neurologic injury presenting as lower extremity numbness. The neurologic involvement may be at the level of the nerve root(s), the lumbosacral plexus, or even the peripheral nerves (most commonly sciatic nerve). Examples of pelvic ring injuries most frequently associated with neurologic deficits include sacral fractures, sacroiliac joint disruptions, and fracture-dislocations of the acetabulum. Although patients with pelvic trauma may exhibit bilateral lower extremity neurologic involvement, it is more common for a single leg to be involved. The treatment of pelvic ring injuries is discussed in detail in Chapter 28.

Trauma to the lower extremity may involve injury to one or more peripheral nerves. A variety of dislocations and fractures in the lower extremity may be responsible for the neurologic deficit. The initial step in the management of these patients involves the appropriate treatment for the associated skeletal injury. Dislocations must be reduced expeditiously and fractures immobilized or stabilized. The neurologic injuries then are managed expectantly, with the prognosis for recovery of function dependent on the extent of neurologic injury. If injury to the common peroneal or deep peroneal nerves is identified, the leg and ankle should be maintained in a foot drop splint to assist with ambulation and prevent equinus contracture of the ankle while neurologic recovery is awaited.

Patients occasionally may present with peripheral nerve injury in the lower extremity in the absence of skeletal injury. Direct injury to the peripheral nerves is most common with lacerations or penetrating injuries to the leg. If the nerve is completely transected, the prognosis for recovery of function is poor. Results of nerve repair and grafting in the lower extremity generally have not been good. As a final note regarding peripheral nerve injuries in the lower extremity, excellent function can be anticipated with isolated injury to the saphenous or sural nerves in the hind foot because these nerves have no motor function.

If compartment syndrome of the thigh or leg is responsible for the disturbance in lower extremity sensibility, emergent fasciotomy is indicated. The physician should remember, however, that numbness is a relatively late finding in compartment syndrome, and muscle damage may be irreversible. Compartment syndromes are discussed in more detail in Chapter 32.

PROBLEMS PARTICULAR
TO CHILDREN

36

PRINCIPLES OF PEDIATRIC FRACTURE CARE

CHILDREN ARE NOT SIMPLY SMALL ADULTS

William T. Obremskey

■ ANATOMIC DIFFERENCES

The major difference between the skeletons of children and adults is that children's bones have physes (growth plates). Bones in children are growing, constantly changing structures, with most longitudinal growth occurring at the physes at the proximal and distal ends of most long bones. When subjected to traumatic forces, bones, like chains, fail at their weakest link; in a child's bone, that weak link is the physis. Also, because the periosteum is thicker and stronger in children than in adults, fractures in children generally exhibit less deformity, are more stable following closed reduction, and heal more rapidly than those in adults.

■ BIOMECHANICAL DIFFERENCES

Bones in children are less dense than those in adults, primarily because of greater porosity caused by a greater number of blood vessels within the cortex of the bone. This greater porosity allows a child's bone to bend, undergo plastic deformation, and be subject to compression fractures. A fracture in compression commonly is called a buckle or a torus fracture (Fig. 36–1A), a term that comes from the resemblance of the fracture to a raised band around the base of an architectural column.

Bones in children bend before they break, and if the bending force is released before actual fracturing occurs, some residual bend will remain in the bone. This residual bend is called plastic deformation and is seen most commonly in the ulna and the fibula (Fig. 36–1B). If the bone is bent beyond its ability to undergo plastic deformation, a greenstick fracture may occur. A greenstick fracture (incomplete fracture) disrupts the side of the bone that is in tension but does not extend all the way across to the other side of the bone, which is in compression. If even greater energy is transmitted to a child's bone, a complete fracture will result, as occurs in adult bones.

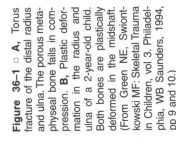

Figure 36–1 □ **A,** Torus fracture of the distal radius and ulna. The porous metaphyseal bone fails in compression. **B,** Plastic deformation in the radius and ulna of a 2-year-old child. Both bones are plastically deformed in the midshaft. (From Green NE, Swiontkowski MF: Skeletal Trauma in Children, vol 3. Philadelphia, WB Saunders, 1994, pp 9 and 10.)

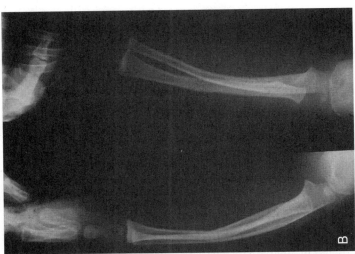

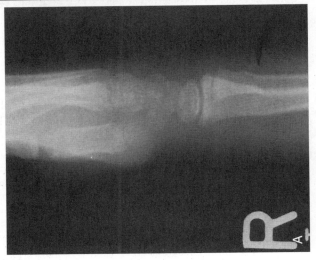

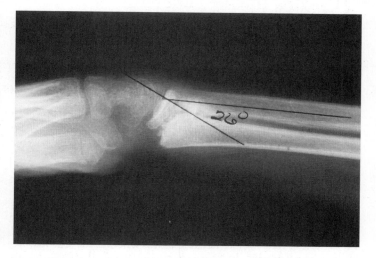

Figure 36–2 □ Lateral radiograph of a distal radial fracture with apex volar angulation in a 9-year-old child. This deformity was completely remodeled in 6 months.

■ PHYSIOLOGIC DIFFERENCES

The remaining longitudinal growth in the bones of children enables them to correct angular deformities resulting from fractures. Fractures occurring near joints and in which the fracture angulation is in the plane of the motion of the joint have the greatest capacity for remodeling. For example, fractures of the distal radius with dorsal or volar angulation will remodel extensively, since the deformity is in the plane of wrist flexion and extension (Fig. 36–2). Fractures in long bones often stimulate excessive growth, probably because of the enhanced blood flow associated with fracture healing. This is seen commonly in fractures of the femur, where there may be 1 to 2 cm of excess growth to compensate for shortening at the fracture site.

A fracture through the physis of a long bone can result in arrested growth. Physeal arrest may lead to decreased longitudinal growth, malformation of the adjacent articular surface, or angular deformity. Physiologically, children's fractures heal much more rapidly than do those in adults because of the abundant blood flow to the bone and periosteum. The plasticity of the bones, the thickened periosteum, and the speed of healing allow most fractures in children to be treated successfully by nonsurgical methods.

■ PHYSEAL FRACTURES

Fractures through the physis make up approximately one third of extremity fractures in children. The cells that account for longitudinal growth of the bone reside in the physis. Because of the potential for disturbances of growth, all children with physeal fractures with any displacement are best referred to an orthopaedist for management.

The Salter-Harris classification system of physeal fractures is generally accepted (Fig. 36–3). In this classification system, the higher the numeric class of the fracture, the greater the energy required to produce the injury and the higher the risk of growth arrest. In *Salter-Harris I fractures* the fracture line passes only through the physeal growth plate. In general, these fractures occur with a low level of trauma and have a low incidence of growth arrest. Children with normal radiographs but who have tenderness over the physis of a bone most likely have a Salter-Harris I fracture and are best managed with immobilization. If the diagnosis is unclear, stress radiographs may be taken to assess whether there is opening of the injured physis. In *Salter-Harris II fractures* the fracture line

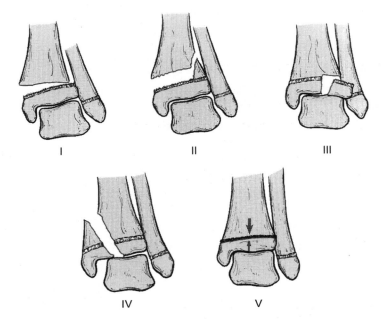

Figure 36–3 □ The Salter-Harris classification of physeal injury (see text for explanation). (From Green NE, Swiontkowski MF: Skeletal Trauma in Children, vol 3. Philadelphia, WB Saunders, 1994, p 20.)

passes through the physis and exits through the adjacent metaphysis. Usually these fractures are reduced easily by nonoperative methods and are associated with a low incidence of growth arrest. In *Salter-Harris III fractures* the fracture line passes through the physis and exits through the epiphysis into the joint. It is generally accepted that management of these fractures requires nearly anatomic reduction of the articular surface. In *Salter-Harris IV fractures* the fracture line begins in the metaphysis, extends through the physis, and exits into the joint through the epiphysis. The intraarticular component of this injury needs to be accurately reduced and stabilized until union occurs. This type of fracture most commonly is seen about the ankle and elbow in children whose growth plates are beginning to close. A *Salter-Harris V fracture* is a crushing injury with damage to the germinal cells of the physis; these fractures carry a high risk of growth arrest.

■ SUMMARY

Children's bones are anatomically different from adult bones; children's bones have a physis, where bone growth is occurring, and a thick periosteum, which imparts stability and is capable of rapid new bone formation. Unlike the brittle long bones of adults, those of children may undergo plastic deformation and sustain compression and greenstick fractures. The physiology of children's bones allows for a great deal of remodeling following periarticular fractures, as well as for overgrowth of diaphyseal fractures, particularly in the femur. The growth potential of a child's bone, however, can also result in progressive deformity following fractures involving the growth plate.

Growth plate injuries occur only in children with open physes. The Salter-Harris classification provides an accurate and simple description of these fractures. Most physeal fractures can be managed nonoperatively with a low risk of growth plate arrest. Crushing injuries to the physis, however, have a high incidence of growth plate arrest. Intraarticular physeal fractures require nearly anatomic realignment and possibly internal stabilization. If the deformity is progressive, surgical treatment may be required to correct it and improve function.

37

OSTEOMYELITIS
AND SEPTIC ARTHRITIS

William T. Obremskey

Osteomyelitis and septic arthritis are seen much more commonly in children than in adults. Experimental data have shown that osteomyelitis and septic arthritis most frequently are caused by bacteremia coupled with local trauma, two circumstances common in childhood. The metaphyses of the fast growing bones of children seem to be predisposed to bacterial infection because of the low flow state of the blood circulation and the diminished phagocytosis of bacteria in this region. In children less than 12 to 18 months of age, metaphyseal osteomyelitis can cross the physis and enter the epiphysis, whereas this does not occur in older children.

Early treatment of osteomyelitis and septic arthritis is imperative to avoid long-term complications. Delayed diagnosis and treatment of osteomyelitis can result in injury to a growth plate and growth arrest, and untreated septic arthritis can irreversibly damage the articular cartilage.

Bone and joint infections commonly are confused with tumors. Diaphyseal osteomyelitis commonly is confused with Ewing's sarcoma or neuroblastoma. Metaphyseal osteomyelitis can be confused with osteogenic sarcoma or an acute fracture of the growth plate. Septic arthritis can be confused with monoarticular juvenile rheumatoid arthritis (JRA). Early septic arthritis of the hip joint can be difficult to differentiate from toxic synovitis.

■ PHONE CALL

Questions

1. How old is the patient?

The patient's age can be an important clue in identifying the infecting organism. In the neonate the most common infecting organisms are group B streptococci, *Escherichia coli,* and *Staphylococcus aureus.* In children under 4 years of age, common pathogens are *Haemophilus influenzae, S. aureus,* and streptococci. In otherwise healthy children 4 years of age and older, *S. aureus* is the infecting organism in about 90% of cases (Table 37–1).

Table 37–1 □ **COMMONLY ISOLATED ORGANISMS IN MONOMICROBIAL OSTEOMYELITIS ACCORDING TO AGE OF THE PATIENT**

Infant (<1 y)	Child (1–16 y)	Adult (>16 y)
Group B streptococci *Staphylococcus aureus* *Escherichia coli*	*Staphylococcus aureus* *Streptococcus pyogenes* *Haemophilus influenzae*	*Staphylococcus aureus* *Staphylococcus epidermidis* *Pseudomonas aeruginosa* *Serratia marcescens* *Escherichia coli*

2. **How long have the symptoms been present?**
   Osteomyelitis and septic arthritis usually are characterized by a fairly acute onset, whereas tumors of bone usually are characterized by a more insidious onset of symptoms.
3. **Has the patient sustained an injury?**
   Osteomyelitis and septic arthritis seem to be associated with a recent injury in about 40% to 60% of children. In animal studies, bacteremia itself did not result in osteomyelitis, but bacteremia combined with local trauma resulted in osteomyelitis in nearly all cases. A Salter-Harris fracture also can mimic a bone or joint infection.
4. **Does the child have an underlying medical condition?**
   Children who are immunocompromised because of cancer treatment, human immunodeficiency virus (HIV) infection, or other immune disorders are susceptible to opportunistic infections. A flare of JRA or the initial onset of JRA can mimic a bone or joint infection. A thrombotic crisis in sickle cell disease can be difficult to differentiate from a bone or joint infection.
5. **Is the patient febrile?**
   Fever may be helpful in indicating infection as opposed to other diagnoses. The physician must remember, however, that only about 25% of patients with osteomyelitis or septic arthritis have a fever.

Orders

Laboratory.   CBC, ESR, and C-reactive protein (CRP).

X-ray.   AP and lateral radiographs of the involved extremity. Radiographs often are not helpful in acute osteomyelitis since the radiographic changes of osteomyelitis take 7 to 10 days to become evident. Radiographs will, however, generally rule out fracture or bone tumor.

Inform RN

"I will arrive at the bedside/emergency department in 15 to 30 minutes." Unless the child is in septic shock, osteomyelitis is not a true emergency; nonetheless, any child with suspected osteomyelitis should be evaluated urgently. Septic arthritis can irreversibly damage articular cartilage in less than 24 hours. This is especially true in the pediatric hip joint.

■ ELEVATOR THOUGHTS

Affections of Joints
- Inflammatory
  Transient synovitis of the hip (toxic synovitis)
  Pyogenic arthritis
  Tuberculous arthritis
  Fungal arthritis
  Juvenile rheumatoid arthritis

Affections of Bone
- Inflammatory
  Acute and chronic osteomyelitis
- Neoplastic
  Osteogenic sarcoma
  Ewing's sarcoma
  Eosinophilic granuloma
- Congenital
  Osteogenesis imperfecta with periarticular fractures
  Congenital insensitivity to pain with periarticular fractures
- Metabolic
  Sickle cell disease with thrombotic crisis

■ BEDSIDE

Vital Signs

Vital signs should be taken for any child with suspected osteomyelitis or septic arthritis. An elevated temperature is seen in only 25% of children with bone or joint infections, but a fever is more likely to be seen with an infection than with a bone tumor or fracture

Selective History

What is the duration of the pain?
An infectious cause is commonly heralded by 1 to 3 days of severe pain. Low-grade pain over several weeks is more consistent with a bone tumor.

Has the child been able to use the extremity?

When an infection develops, a child generally will quit using an extremity voluntarily. In many cases the earliest sign of osteomyelitis or septic arthritis in the lower limb is that the child refuses to walk on the involved limb.

What is the exact location of pain?

Although many children are unable to precisely localize their pain, the site of maximal pain, if it can be determined, is the most likely site of infection.

Selective Physical Examination

Inspection

The physician should inspect the painful limb for erythema and edema. The physician also should observe how the child uses the involved extremity. If the child can walk on the affected lower limb or can use the affected upper limb for grasping and other activities, it is not likely to be infected. The physician also should observe the resting position of the extremity. For example, in septic arthritis of the hip the limb usually will be held in a flexed and externally rotated position; this position relaxes the hip capsule and may somewhat decrease the intraarticular pressure generated by the septic arthritis.

Palpation

Every square centimeter of the involved extremity should be palpated to identify the point of maximum tenderness. Identifying the point of maximum tenderness is helpful in directed aspiration (if needed) to obtain cultures and guide treatment. The joints of the affected limb should also be palpated for effusion. An effusion may be a primary effusion resulting from septic arthritis, or it may be a reactive effusion due to nearby infection or inflammation. Any joint suspected of being infected should be aspirated, and the aspirate sent for culture.

Movement

Passive and active range of motion of the extremity should be assessed. Children with periarticular osteomyelitis or septic arthritis usually are resistant to movement of the involved extremity. With infection, pain usually is severe and the child strongly resists any movement of the limb.

■ FURTHER ORDERS

Plain radiographs are often inconclusive but should be obtained to rule out chronic infection, fracture, or tumor. If the diagnosis is in doubt, a bone scan can be obtained. Bone scans are highly sensitive but nonspecific: they cannot differentiate between sepsis, tumor, and injury. A bone scan is most helpful in evaluating for possible osteomyelitis in the pelvis and thoracolumbar spine, areas not easily accessed for physical examination.

Cultures may be obtained from the blood, bone, or joint. Blood cultures and aspirates of an infected bone or joint are positive in approximately 60% of children with bone infection. If both blood cultures and bone aspiration are performed, the organism is identified in about 80% of cases of bone infection. Aspiration of bone is performed at the site of maximal tenderness on the involved extremity. The material aspirated from the bone or joint should be sent for culture and sensitivity. The joint aspirate should also be sent for cell count and microscopic analysis for the presence of crystals (Table 37–1). An aspirate with a total white blood cell count of 80,000 to 100,000/ml is highly indicative of an infectious process.

■ MANAGEMENT

All patients with suspected osteomyelitis or septic arthritis should be admitted to the hospital for evaluation. If a diagnosis of osteomyelitis is made (either after aspiration and Gram stain or purely based on the history and symptoms), intravenous antibiotics should be started immediately. If pus is encountered upon aspiration of the bone but it is believed the abscess was significantly relieved with the aspiration, the patient may be managed with intravenous antibiotics alone. If the child does not greatly improve in approximately 72 hours, serious consideration must be given to surgical debridement of the involved area.

Children with septic arthritis should be treated with intravenous antibiotics. Additional surgical treatment may involve serial aspirations for reaccumulation of fluid in the joint or surgical irrigation and debridement. The only exception is the hip joint, which always requires open surgical irrigation and debridement, since there is a high risk of avascular necrosis or of chondral damage to the femoral head if the hip is not surgically drained.

The appropriate initial antibiotic is age dependent, since patients in different age groups tend to be infected with different organisms (Table 37–1). Neonates are at greatest risk for infection due to group B streptococci, *S. aureus,* and *E. coli.* These patients should be treated with a semisynthetic, beta-lactamase-resistant penicillin and an aminoglycoside or with a third-generation cephalosporin. Antibiotic recommendations rarely stay the same, so it is best if the physician follows the antibiotic recommendations in his or her hospital. Suggested initial antibiotic therapy is listed in Table 37–2.

Table 37–2 □ **INITIAL ANTIBIOTIC THERAPY FOR OSTEOMYELITIS IN CHILDREN**

Initial Antibiotic Choice	Comment
Oxacillin 150 mg/kg per 24 h	*Staphylococcus aureus* suspected infecting organism
Cefazolin 100 mg/kg	If allergic to penicillins
Clindamycin 25 mg/kg per 24 h *or*	If allergic to both penicillins and cephalosporins
Vancomycin 40 mg/kg per 24 h	

The duration of treatment has been controversial. Classically, children received antibiotics intravenously for six weeks. This "magic number" comes from reports of a higher incidence of recurrent infection in children who received less than 28 days of adequate treatment. Most current regimens consist of 3 to 7 days of intravenous antibiotic therapy, followed by 4 to 6 weeks of appropriate oral antibiotics, as determined by the results of the bone or joint fluid cultures. The decision to switch to oral antibiotics is based on the child's clinical response to intravenous therapy and the isolation of an organism sensitive to an oral agent. The choice of oral agent should be dictated by the results of culture and sensitivities. Commonly used agents are listed in Table 37–3. Blood levels of the oral antibiotics may be measured to assure compliance and to ascertain whether they are high enough to be bactericidal.

Special Situations

The Neonate

The advent of neonatal intensive care units and the survival of greater numbers of premature infants have led to an increase in infections among neonates. Neonates and premature infants have an immature immune system that limits their inflammatory response to a bone or joint infection, making detection difficult. Neonates with bone or joint infections may manifest no clinical signs other

Table 37–3 □ **COMMONLY USED ORAL ANALGESICS IN THE TREATMENT OF OSTEOMYELITIS IN CHILDREN**

Agent	Dose
Cephalexin	150 mg/kg per 24 h
Clindamycin	50 mg/kg per 24 h
Dicloxacillin	50 mg/kg

than irritability. Therefore, if a bone or joint infection is suspected in a neonate, the suspected locus should be aspirated and the fluid sent for Gram stain and culture. It is important not to delay aspiration or treatment while awaiting further clinical signs of a particular focus of infection, since joints can be destroyed rapidly by an untreated infection. Because of the many invasive procedures performed on premature infants, a wide variety of infectious organisms can be found in these patients. The most common organism is group B streptococci, but there is also a high incidence of *S. aureus.* Opportunistic organisms, such as *Candida albicans,* also need to be considered as potential pathogens.

Sickle Cell Disease

Children with sickle cell anemia are at high risk for developing osteomyelitis. Infection commonly is due to *Salmonella* or staphylococci, but infection due to either one can be difficult to differentiate from a thrombotic crisis. The signs and symptoms of osteomyelitis and thrombotic crisis essentially are the same and usually include a mild fever, tenderness to palpation over the bones, and a relatively acute onset of symptoms. Bone scans and MRI scans generally are not helpful in distinguishing bone infarction from osteomyelitis.

It is important to make a prompt diagnosis and to begin treatment. Patients should be treated initially as if they are having a thrombotic crisis, but in addition bones that are focally tender should be aspirated for specimens for Gram stain and bacterial culture. Empiric treatment with antibiotics should be based on the overall clinical picture of the patient or the presence of pus on aspiration.

Diskitis

Diskitis has a spectrum of presentations, ranging from mild inflammation in a younger child to acute osteomyelitis in adolescence. It has been debated whether diskitis is actually an infectious process because in younger children it often has a self-limiting course when managed with bed rest and bracing. It is now generally accepted, however, that diskitis is a result of an infectious process. The possibility of diskitis can be overlooked easily in a young child who presents with irritability, fatigue, or refusal to walk. Older children usually present with back pain, abdominal pain, and fatigue. Radiographic changes are not present for 2 to 3 weeks and consist of narrowing of the disk space and erosion of the end plates of the vertebral bodies. A technetium bone scan may be positive within the first several days, however. Cultures of peripheral venous blood and biopsy material are positive in less than 50% of children with diskitis. Because of the low incidence of positive cultures, a biopsy is not indicated unless the child does not respond to intravenous antibiotics. Children with diskitis initially should be treated with intravenous antibiotics to cover *S. aureus*, the most common infectious agent, and then may be changed to oral antibiotics when their condition improves. *Mycobacterium tuberculosis* and *Coccidioides immitis* (coccidioidomycosis) also should be considered as potential pathogens in children who do not respond to antistaphylococcal therapy.

Puncture Wounds

Although common, puncture wounds in the feet of children only rarely result in osteomyelitis. The usual history is one of a child wearing tennis shoes stepping on a nail and receiving initial treatment in the local emergency room with local irrigation and a tetanus shot. It is estimated that only 8% of patients treated this way will develop cellulitis, treatable with antistaphylococcal antibiotics. Deep puncture wounds over the metatarsal heads or the calcaneus, however, have a high likelihood of penetrating bone, resulting in osteomyelitis, most commonly caused by *Pseudomonas*. In these instances the physician should consider early, deep wound debridement and treatment with an antipseudomonal agent.

38

DEVELOPMENTAL HIP DYSPLASIA

William T. Obremskey

Developmental dysplasia of the hip (DDH), a condition that indicates an abnormally developing acetabulum, is seen in newborns and young children. This condition previously was called congenital hip dysplasia, but the name was changed to reflect the possibility of hips being normal at birth but becoming dysplastic over time. Hip dysplasia is caused by a combination of genetic and positional factors. The incidence of DDH is approximately 1.5/1000 live births in whites and 0.5/1000 live births in blacks. Girls are at greater risk for developing DDH. The incidence is 1.1/1000 live births in females and 0.1/1000 live births in males. A family history of hip dysplasia further increases a child's risk. Positional factors in pregnancy, such as breech presentation and oligohydramnios, also can lead to a higher incidence of DDH. The underlying problem in DDH is that the femoral head is not deeply seated in the acetabulum, causing the acetabulum to be shallow and incompletely developed. The disorder has a spectrum of presentations, ranging from a shallow acetabulum to completely dislocated hips. It is important to identify and treat DDH early, as outcomes improve the earlier treatment is initiated.

The long-term consequences of untreated DDH can be devastating. A child with a poorly developed acetabulum can be expected to have hip pain and limited function in early adulthood. A child with completely dislocated hips that go untreated will have significant pain with walking, a waddling gait, low back pain, and ipsilateral knee pain.

■ PHONE CALL

Questions

1. How old is the patient?

The younger the patient at initiation of treatment, the more likely nonoperative treatment will be successful.

2. What is the child's sex?

Girls have a higher incidence of DDH than boys do.

3. Were there any problems associated with pregnancy and birth?

It is important to know if the mother had oligohydramnios, if the child was in a breech position, or if the child had a traumatic birth.

4. Is there a family history of DDH?

A mother who had a history of hip dysplasia as a child has a higher risk of having a female child with hip dysplasia. An older sibling with DDH also increases a child's risk of having DDH.

5. What is the child's ethnicity?

The incidence of DDH is greater in whites and some native Americans.

Orders

None.

Inform RN

"I will arrive at the bedside sometime today." Hip dysplasia is not an emergency, but the earlier treatment is initiated, the more likely it will be successful. Newborns with a reliable family can be seen as outpatients within a week of hospital discharge for examination, possible imaging, and discussion of treatment options.

■ ELEVATOR THOUGHTS

- Injuries
    Femur fractures due to birth trauma
- Infection
    Pyogenic arthritis (especially in a child in the neonatal intensive care unit)
- Associated conditions
    Arthrogryposis
    Congenital muscular torticollis
    Metatarsus adductus

■ BEDSIDE

Vital Signs

None.

Selective History

Is the child the firstborn?
What is the child's sex?
Was the child born breech?
Did the mother have oligohydramnios during pregnancy?
Is there a family history of DDH?
Did other siblings have DDH?

Each of the preceding factors is associated with a higher incidence of DDH.

Selective Physical Examination

Inspection

A newborn with DDH will have no obvious physical abnormalities. An older child will have extra thigh folds on the side of the DDH and apparent shortening of the involved femur. An older child also will have a shortened femur if the hips and knees are flexed 90 degrees. This is called Galeazzi sign (Fig. 38–1) .

Testing

The examination of a crying newborn for DDH can be difficult. DDH is much easier to detect in a relaxed feeding or sleeping infant. Testing the newborn infant is best done with the child on a firm surface in the supine position. The hips are flexed to 90 degrees. The knee is cupped in the first web space of the examiner's hand, with the thumb placed medially. The long and ring fingers are then placed just beneath the greater trochanter of the proximal femur. One leg is held still and the other leg is gently abducted while the long and ring fingers gently lift the trochanter upward. Feeling a "clunk of reduction" is a positive Ortolani sign. The thigh is adducted while the examiner gently presses down with the palm of the hand. Feeling a dislocation or "clunk" is a positive Barlow sign. The examiner should note the range of abduction in which the hip is stable in the acetabulum (Fig. 38–2).

A dislocated hip in an older child frequently cannot be reduced. On physical examination the physician will note a shortened femur and extra thigh folds on the involved side. Older children also may have limited abduction on the involved side.

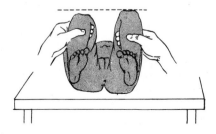

Figure 38–1 □ The Galeazzi sign: apparent shortening of the femur on the side with the dislocated hip. (From Tachdjian MO: Pediatric Orthopedics, 2nd ed. Philadelphia, WB Saunders, 1990, p 326.)

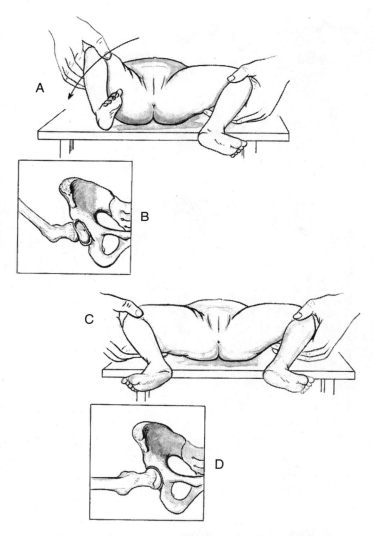

Figure 38–2 □ The Ortolani test (see text for description). The Barlow test is the reverse of the Ortolani test. (From Tachdjian MO: Pediatric Orthopedics, 2nd ed. Philadelphia, WB Saunders, 1990, p 313.)

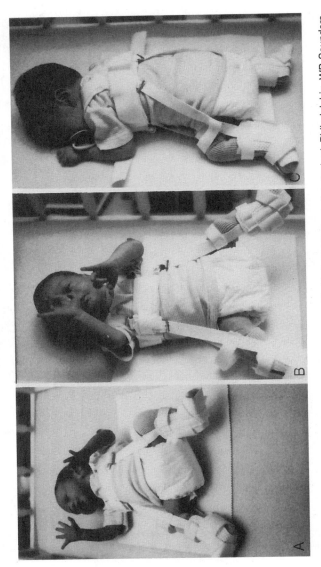

Figure 38–3 □ The Pavlik harness. (From Tachdjian MO: Pediatric Orthopedics, 2nd ed. Philadelphia, WB Saunders, 1990, p 331.)

■ FURTHER ORDERS

If the examination indicates DDH, the physician should order an AP radiograph of the pelvis with the legs symmetrically adducted and the hips flexed approximately 30 degrees. Children who have an examination that does not indicate DDH but who previously had an examination with a questionable result may need a follow-up radiograph in 4 to 6 weeks and a repeat examination. If that examination is inconclusive, ultrasonography can be used to aid in identifying any hip dysplasia.

■ MANAGEMENT

Ideally DDH is diagnosed and treated initially in the newborn period by an orthopaedic specialist. The standard current treatment is a Pavlik harness. The harness is placed on the child so that it holds the legs at approximately 100 degrees of flexion and in some abduction (Fig. 38–3). A child with unstable hips *should not* be removed from the Pavlik harness by the parent, and the child should have follow-up visits on a weekly basis to assure maintenance of adequate reduction. The length of treatment necessary in a Pavlik harness varies with the severity of the dysplasia, but as a general rule, treatment time in the harness is 6 weeks plus 1 week for every week of age the child was at the time of diagnosis.

Radiographic or ultrasound evaluation should be obtained immediately after placing the child in the Pavlik harness to assure concentric reduction of the femoral heads in the acetabulum. A follow-up radiographic or ultrasound examination should be done in approximately 4 weeks to assure maintenance of reduction.

The child who is diagnosed with a subluxatable or dislocated hip at 6 months of age or greater should be referred immediately to an orthopaedic specialist.

39

INITIAL MANAGEMENT
OF CLUBFOOT

William T. Obremskey

Clubfoot is one of the earliest described congenital birth deformities. This foot deformity has a wide spectrum of presentations, but in general the ankle is plantar flexed, the heel inverted, and the forefoot supinated, hence the name *talipes equinovarus*. Although most clubfeet occur in otherwise normal infants, the deformity can be seen in several rare syndromes and neuropathies or myopathies. The overall incidence of talipes equinovarus is 1.24/1000 live births. There does seem to be a heritable component to the condition: the incidence in first-degree relatives of affected children is much higher than in the general population. The cause of the clubfoot deformity has not been determined precisely, although several theories have been offered.

■ PHONE CALL

Questions

1. **How old is the patient?**

    Talipes equinovarus is present at birth. Foot deformities occurring after birth should lead the physician to suspect conditions other than clubfoot. Although clubfoot occurs with a wide range of severity, in general the earlier the treatment, the better the prognosis.

2. **Is there a family history of clubfeet?**

    Although not yet proven, there seems to be a heritable component to talipes equinovarus.

3. **Are there other associated syndromes or birth defects?**

    Any child with one congenital deformity should be carefully examined for other deformities. Although most clubfeet occur in isolation, the condition occasionally is associated with other deformities, which should be sought (see Elevator Thoughts).

4. **Were there problems during pregnancy such as oligohydramnios?**

    Abnormalities during pregnancy, such as oligohydramnios or congenital constriction bands, have been associated with a higher incidence of clubfeet.

Orders

None.

Inform RN

"I will arrive at the bedside or emergency department within 24 hours." The outcome following treatment of a clubfoot is best if treatment begins early in the child's life. The child may be seen in an orthopaedic clinic within a week of discharge from the hospital. When possible, however, it is desirable to have an orthopaedist speak with the child's family before the child leaves the hospital. The birth of a child with a congenital deformity often causes great anxiety in the parents, and early counseling by an orthopaedist as to the expected treatment and its outcome can often help allay the family's fears.

■ ELEVATOR THOUGHTS

Causes of Talipes Equinovarus
- Oligohydramnios
- Constriction band
- Genetic causes
    Freeman-Sheldon syndrome (whistling face syndrome, craniocarpotarsal dystrophy)
    Diastrophic dwarfism
    Larsen's syndrome
    Smith-Lemli-Optiz syndrome
    Goldenhar's syndrome
- Neuropathies or myopathies with myelodysplasia
    Cerebral palsy
    Arthrogryposis
    Spinal muscular atrophy and muscular dystrophy

■ BEDSIDE

Vital Signs

None needed.

Selective History

What is the child's age?
    Although the diagnosis of talipes equinovarus is usually made at birth, the physician occasionally will encounter older patients with clubfoot that has not been treated. Treatment is much more difficult in these patients.

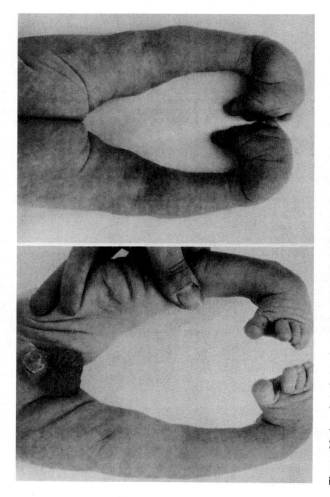

Figure 39–1 □ Anterior and posterior views of clubfoot in a newborn infant. Note the inversion of the hindfeet and varus of the forefeet. (From Tachdjian MO: Pediatric Orthopedics, 2nd ed. Philadelphia, WB Saunders, 1990, p 2449.)

What is the child's sex?
Clubfoot is seen more often in boys than in girls.

Are there associated congenital abnormalities?
Clubfoot associated with other congenital anomalies, such as arthrogryposis, is much more resistant to treatment than is isolated clubfoot.

Is there any family history of clubfoot?
See chapter opening discussion.

Did the mother have oligohydramnios during pregnancy?
See Question 4.

Selective Physical Examination

Inspection

The entire leg should be inspected and compared to the other leg. Atrophy of the calf commonly is seen in clubfoot, and shortening of the entire limb occasionally is seen. There is a medial crease, and the lateral border of the foot is curved (Fig. 39–1). In severe cases the child may have a cavus deformity (extremely high medial longitudinal arch).

Palpation

It is important to determine the range of movement of the knee and ankle, as well as the flexibility of the foot deformity. Flexible deformities that can be corrected easily with stretching are more amenable to nonoperative treatment than are fixed deformities. Marked stiffness of the knee and ankle may be a sign of arthrogryposis.

■ FURTHER ORDERS

Simulated-weight-bearing AP and lateral radiographs of the foot should be obtained. Weight bearing is simulated by pressing the sole of the child's foot against a flat surface, positioning the ankle in maximal dorsiflexion. These radiographs allow determination of the severity of the bony deformity.

■ MANAGEMENT

All children with talipes equinovarus should be referred to an orthopaedist for treatment. The initial management of all idiopathic clubfeet is stretching and casting. This should be done by an orthopaedist familiar with the treatment of clubfeet and should begin in the hospital nursery or outpatient clinic in the first week of life. Before the child is seen by an orthopaedic surgeon, the child's family may be taught how to perform stretching exercises to try to straighten the foot as much as possible. These exercises include attempting to dorsiflex the ankle by pushing up on the mid-aspect of the foot and bending the forefoot out of adduction. Stretching should be gentle and steady and should be performed several times a day.

When managed by an orthopaedist, the foot is stretched for 5 to 10 minutes, and then an above-the-knee cast is applied with the knee in 90-degree flexion and the foot in the maximally corrected position. Casts are changed at 1- to 2-week intervals, depending on the degree of deformity of the clubfoot and the ability of the child to withstand the cast. Even if the clubfoot cannot be completely corrected with casting, casting stretches the skin and soft tissue structures in the foot to make surgical release easier. Clubfeet refractory to stretching and casting should be surgically corrected by an orthopaedic surgeon trained in this deformity and its management.

40

ORTHOPAEDIC ISSUES
IN HEMOPHILIA

William T. Obremskey

Hemophilia is a bleeding disorder caused by a congenital deficiency of clotting factors VIII or IX. The incidence of hemophilia is approximately 10 per 100,000 in the United States, and the ratio of hemophilic patients with factor VIII deficiency to those with factor IX deficiency is 5:1. Hemophilia is inherited as a sex-linked recessive trait. The acute orthopaedic manifestations of hemophilia primarily involve intraarticular and intramuscular bleeding.

Intraarticular and intramuscular bleeding in patients with hemophilia should be treated urgently to control pain and to prevent nerve injury and late fibrosis and contracture. Prevention is important, as repeated hemarthroses or muscle bleeds may lead to fibrosis and nerve injury in the muscle compartment.

■ **PHONE CALL**

Questions

1. **How old is the patient?**

   Intramuscular and intraarticular bleeding are seen commonly in hemophilic patients from the time the child begins to walk until he or she is about 7 years of age, probably because of the high level of activity and frequency of falls in young children. The frequency of severe bleeds usually decreases throughout the teenage years. Patients who have had numerous hemarthroses tend to have less frequent and less severe bleeds over time because of the joint fibrosis, stiffness, and contracture that have ensued.

2. **What is the patient's current level of clotting factors?**

   The magnitude of the clotting factor deficiency can give the physician clues as to the anticipated severity of the bleed, as well as to the expected difficulty in controlling the bleeding. Factor level assays report the percentage of the normally expected factor level in the patient's blood. Factor levels less than 5% are generally seen in hemophilic children with frequent severe bleeds.

3. **Is there an inhibitor?**

   Patients with hemophilia who have received numerous infusions of clotting factor to control bleeding can develop inhibitors (antibodies) to factors VIII or IX. A high titer of inhibitor makes it much more difficult to control bleeding with factor infusions, often changes the medical treatment of the bleeding disorder, and makes invasive management of hemarthroses much less desirable and successful.

4. Is the patient HIV positive?

Patients with hemophilia who have received numerous transfusions of clotting factors are at much greater risk for acquiring the HIV virus than is the general population. Children with AIDS and hemophilia also have a much higher risk of developing septic arthritis, which may mimic a hemarthrosis.

Orders

AP and lateral radiographs of the involved joint or limb should be ordered to rule out fracture as the cause of bleeding into a joint or muscle. In patients who have had numerous hemarthroses, profound osteopenia often develops in the involved limb, placing it at high risk of fracture.

A CBC and ESR also should be ordered, especially if infection is suspected. If a serum level of the child's deficient clotting factor has not been obtained recently, one should be ordered. The level of clotting factor, as well as the titer of an inhibitor, if present, may help guide treatment.

Inform RN

"I will arrive at the bedside/emergency department within 30 minutes." Hemarthroses and intramuscular bleeding should be managed urgently to relieve pain and help prevent complications.

■ ELEVATOR THOUGHTS

- Bleeding disorders
  Hemophilia A (factor VIII deficiency)
  Hemophilia B (factor IX deficiency)
- Inflammations/infections
  Septic arthritis
- Trauma
  Periarticular fractures
- Tumors
  Pseudotumor

■ BEDSIDE

Vital Signs

The child's temperature should be obtained. A fever may indicate a joint infection, and many children with an acute hemarthrosis also are febrile.

Selective History

It is important to know the precise cause of the patient's bleeding disorder (i.e., factor VIII or factor IX deficiency) and whether an inhibitor has developed. Also, the physician must ascertain the location of the involved joint and the duration of pain in the joint or muscle. The physician should inquire about prior bleeding episodes into joints or muscles, as well as about any recent trauma or general illness.

Selective Physical Examination

Inspection

The symptomatic area should be carefully inspected and compared to the contralateral side, with special attention being paid to any deformity or swelling.

Palpation

Both fracture and hemarthrosis are tender to palpation. A tumor or pseudotumor, however, generally is not tender. A tense joint effusion can occur with an intraarticular bleed, a fracture, or an infection.

Range of Motion

Examination of the involved joint should include active and passive range of motion. In any condition that causes a tense effusion, range of motion of the affected joint will be markedly limited because of pain.

Neurovascular Examination

The distal neurovascular status of extremities that have had multiple bleeds should be assessed for sensory or motor changes that would indicate compression of a nerve. Compression of nerves most commonly is seen with bleeding into the iliopsoas muscle, which can compress the femoral nerve and cause numbness of the anterior thigh. Also seen is intramuscular bleeding into the volar forearm compartment, which can compress the median nerve, resulting in numbness of the radial digits of the hand and pain with motion of the finger flexors.

■ FURTHER ORDERS

No additional tests are necessary if radiographs of the involved joint or limb, CBC, and ESR have been obtained. A hematology consult should be sought if the type of hemophilia has not been definitely diagnosed previously or the presence or absence of inhibitors has not been confirmed.

■ MANAGEMENT

Most intramuscular and intraarticular bleeding in patients with hemophilia can be managed nonoperatively. In general the bleeding can be controlled with infusions of cryoprecipitate or the deficient factor as appropriate. Patients with inhibitors may respond to large amounts of factor replacement to overwhelm the inhibitor and control bleeding. In children with a recent history of multiple bleeds, home treatment with factor replacement has decreased the incidence of intraarticular and intramuscular bleeding. Home therapy in patients with severe factor deficiencies can decrease the frequency of bleeds and the severity of their long-term sequelae.

In addition to treatment with infusion of clotting factors, the joint or extremity in which the bleed has occurred should be immobilized. Application of ice packs and administration of narcotics may help control pain. If a patient has a large, tense hemarthrosis, the joint may be aspirated to relieve pain. Aspiration should be performed only after infusion of clotting factors. Unless the factor has been replaced, the hemarthrosis will reaccumulate rapidly after aspiration and the severe pain will recur because of joint distension. Aspiration of hemarthroses also has been shown to facilitate painless range of motion earlier.

Orthopaedic consultation should be obtained for hemophilic patients with intraarticular or intramuscular bleeds and especially for those with signs of nerve compression. Patients with muscle bleeding and mild nerve compression are managed the same as patients with hemarthroses, with splinting, application of ice, and infusion of clotting factor. The physician can expect a slow resolution of the nerve injury in nearly all cases. Patients with severe limb swelling are at risk for compartmental syndrome, so if there is no resolution of the neurologic symptoms after several hours of monitoring and adequate factor replacement, fasciotomy should be considered. Surgery should be performed in patients with hemophilia only if the factor level can be corrected to greater than 50% of the normal level. Compartmental syndrome is discussed in detail in Chapter 32.

Following an acute hemarthrosis the splint should be removed in 2 to 3 days to begin range of motion exercises, often under the direction of a physical therapist.

A pseudotumor is a rare blood cyst seen in patients with severe hemophilia. This begins as a soft tissue mass in the muscles around a large joint but can extend into and erode the bone. Pseudotumors occasionally may originate in the periosteum of the bone, causing subperiosteal and cortical erosion. They are seen most commonly in the pelvis and about the knee. Management of an enlarging pseudotumor consists of factor replacement, followed by operative evacuation of the cyst.

APPENDIX A

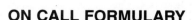

ON CALL FORMULARY

This formulary is a quick reference for information on medications commonly prescribed or administered while the physician is on call. For ease of use, medications are listed alphabetically by generic name under each class of medication; for example, ibuprofen and indomethacin are both included under the broad category of Nonsteroidal Anti-inflammatory Drugs (NSAIDs).

Dosages listed are for adults with normal renal and hepatic function. Antibiotic dosages are listed in Appendix B.

The physician should be aware that many patients require individualization of medication dose. For additional information, the physician should consult the hospital pharmacy or the medication package insert.

ANALGESIC MEDICATIONS

Narcotic Analgesics

Please note that all narcotic analgesic medications may be habit forming and should be used judiciously in patients with musculoskeletal pain. In general, chronic musculoskeletal pain should be treated with nonnarcotic analgesics or NSAIDs.

HYDROCODONE (Vicodin, Vicodin ES, Lortab)

Indications:	Acute pain
Actions:	Narcotic analgesic
Side effects:	Respiratory depression, hypotension, sedation, vomiting, constipation
Dose:	One to two tablets (5–10 mg) PO q4h prn pain

MEPERIDINE (Demerol)

Indications:	Acute pain
Actions:	Narcotic analgesic
Side effects:	Respiratory depression, hypotension, sedation, vomiting, constipation
Dose:	50–150 mg SC/IM/PO q4h prn pain

MORPHINE SULFATE

Indications:	Acute pain
Actions:	Narcotic analgesic
Side effects:	Respiratory depression, hypotension, sedation, vomiting, constipation
Dose:	2–15 mg IM/IV/SC q4h prn pain

OXYCODONE (Percocet, Percodan)

Indications:	Acute pain
Actions:	Narcotic analgesic
Side effects:	Respiratory depression, hypotension, sedation, vomiting, constipation
Dose:	One to two tablets (5–10 mg) PO q4h prn pain

PROPOXYPHENE (Darvocet, Darvon)

Indications:	Acute pain
Actions:	Narcotic analgesic
Side effects:	Respiratory depression, hypotension, sedation, vomiting, constipation
Dose:	100 mg PO q4h prn pain

Nonnarcotic Analgesics

Please note that all NSAIDs (see pp. 313 and 314) have some analgesic activity and that some nonnarcotic analgesic medications may be habit forming (i.e., Ultram).

ACETAMINOPHEN (Tylenol and others)

Indications:	Pain and fever
Actions:	Raises the pain threshold; acts on the hypothalamic heat regulating center
Side effects:	Uncommon—rash, pancytopenia, hepatic toxicity
Dose:	325–1000 mg PO q4h prn, to 4000 mg/24 h

TRAMADOL (Ultram)

Indications:	Pain
Actions:	Binds to opioid receptors; inhibits reuptake of norepinephrine and serotonin
Side effects:	Respiratory depression, hypotension, nausea, constipation
Dose:	50–100 mg PO q6h prn; not to exceed 400 mg/d
Note:	**Has been shown to be habit forming, especially in patients with a previous opioid dependency**

ANESTHETIC MEDICATIONS, LOCAL (FOR INJECTION)

Nearly all local anesthetics are supplied as solutions, either plain or with epinephrine 1/100,000. Solutions containing epinephrine cause local vasoconstriction and, in general, double the duration of action of the anesthetic agent. Local anesthetic solutions containing epinephrine should not be used in anatomic regions where there is no collateral circulation, most notably the fingers, toes, and male genitalia. Use of local anesthetics containing epinephrine in these regions may impede blood flow, causing necrosis distal to the site of injection.

BUPIVACAINE (Marcaine)

Indications:	Minor surgery or diagnostic procedures requiring local anesthesia
Actions:	Local anesthesia
Side effects:	Rare, unless large doses absorbed systemically; nausea, hypotension, confusion, seizures, dizziness
Duration:	3–4 hours
How supplied:	0.25% and 0.5% solutions, with or without epinephrine
Dose:	As needed for adequate local anesthesia of region of interest; total dose administered should not exceed 2 mg/kg

LIDOCAINE (Xylocaine)

Indications:	Minor surgery or diagnostic procedures requiring local anesthesia
Actions:	Local anesthesia
Side effects:	Rare, unless large doses absorbed systemically; nausea, hypotension, confusion, seizures, dizziness
Duration:	1–2 hours
How supplied:	1% and 2% solutions, with or without epinephrine
Dose:	As needed for adequate local anesthesia of region of interest; total dose administered should not exceed 7 mg/kg

ANTISPASMODIC MEDICATIONS

The physician should note that no antispasmodics are truly "muscle relaxants." All medications in this class work centrally to decrease CNS activity; thus all antispasmodics are sedating, and many can be habit forming.

CYCLOBENZAPRINE (Flexeril)

Indications:	As an adjunct to rest and physical therapy for relief of muscle spasm associated with acute musculoskeletal conditions
Actions:	CNS depressant
Side effects:	Drowsiness, dry mouth, dizziness, nausea, headache, blurred vision
Dose:	10 mg PO tid

DIAZEPAM (Valium and others)

Indications:	Relief of skeletal muscle spasm
Actions:	CNS depressant
Side effects:	Drowsiness, fatigue, ataxia, confusion, diplopia, dysarthria
Dose:	2–10 mg IV/IM/PO q4–6h prn

METAXALONE (Skelaxin and others)

Indications:	As an adjunct to rest and physical therapy for relief of muscle spasm associated with acute musculoskeletal conditions
Actions:	Not clearly identified; likely CNS depressant
Side effects:	Nausea, vomiting, drowsiness, dizziness, headache
Dose:	800 mg PO q8h prn

CORTICOSTEROID MEDICATIONS

Injectable

Injectable corticosteroids are used most commonly in musculoskeletal medicine for injection of inflamed joints or bursae. Before injecting a corticosteroid into any area, the physician must be certain there is no infection present. The physician also must be careful not to inject corticosteroid medications directly into tendons, as weakening and possibly rupture of the tendon may result. All injected corticosteroid medications can cause fat necrosis and depigmentation of the skin at the site of injection.

BETAMETHASONE (Celestone)

Indications:	Inflamed joints or bursae
Actions:	Potent anti-inflammatory agent
Side effects:	*Commonly,* increased pain for 24 hours after injection; *uncommonly,* fat necrosis and skin depigmentation at the site of injection; *rarely,* the same side effects as oral corticosteroids (see below)
How supplied:	6 mg/ml suspension
Dose:	0.5–2 ml injected into bursa or joint

METHYLPREDNISOLONE (Depo-Medrol)

Indications:	Inflamed joints or bursae
Actions:	Potent anti-inflammatory agent
Side effects:	*Commonly,* increased pain for 24 hours after injection; *uncommonly,* fat necrosis and skin depigmentation at the site of injection; *rarely,* the same side effects as oral corticosteroids
How supplied:	40 mg/ml and 80 mg/ml suspensions
Dose:	20–80 mg injected into bursa or joint

TRIAMCINOLONE (Aristocort, Aristospan)

Indications:	Inflamed joint or bursae
Actions:	Potent anti-inflammatory agent
Side effects:	*Commonly,* increased pain for 24 hours after injection; *uncommonly,* fat necrosis and skin depigmentation at the site of injection; *rarely,* the same side effects as oral corticosteroids
How supplied:	25 mg/ml suspension (Aristocort); 20 mg/ml suspension (Aristospan)
Dose:	0.5–1 ml injected into joint or bursae

Oral

PREDNISONE (numerous trade names)

Indications:	Short-term adjunctive therapy for inflammatory arthritides, gout, sciatica, acute nonspecific tenosynovitis
Actions:	Potent anti-inflammatory agent
Side effects:	*Rare, for short-term administration;* fluid retention, euphoria, muscle weakness, loss of bone mass, avascular necrosis of bone, gastric ulceration
Dose:	5–60 mg/d; dosage should be individualized, and tapering of dosage prior to discontinuation is recommended

METHYLPREDNISOLONE (Medrol, Medrol Dosepak, and others)

Indications:	Short-term adjunctive therapy for inflammatory arthritides, gout, sciatica, acute nonspecific tenosynovitis
Actions:	Potent anti-inflammatory agent
Side effects:	*Rare, for short-term administration;* fluid retention, euphoria, muscle weakness, loss of bone mass, avascular necrosis of bone, gastric ulceration
Dose:	4–48 mg/d; Medrol Dosepak is a blister pack of methylprednisolone tablets delivering a 6-day taper of the medication; instructions for administration are clearly printed on the package

MEDICATIONS FOR ACUTE ATTACKS OF GOUT

COLCHICINE

Indications:	Acute gouty arthritis
Action:	Unknown (it is not a uricosuric)
Side effects:	Nausea, vomiting, abdominal pain (side effects are dose related)
Dose:	0.6 mg PO/IV q1h until (1) symptoms subside, (2) nausea and vomiting occur, or (3) a total dose of 6 mg is reached; after acute symptoms subside, colchicine may be given for 1 week at a dose of 0.6 mg PO bid.

INDOMETHACIN (Indocin and others)

Please see listing under NSAIDs.

NONSTEROIDAL ANTI-INFLAMMATORY DRUGS (NSAIDs)

Many NSAIDs are currently on the market, and new agents are added each year. The following list contains a few of the commonly used NSAIDs in the acute treatment of musculoskeletal disorders and complaints. For information about additional NSAIDs, the physician is encouraged to consult with the pharmacy at his or her hospital.

ASPIRIN (numerous trade names)

Indications:	Fever, pain due to inflammation
Actions:	Centrally, reduces pain perception; peripherally, interferes with production of prostaglandins
Side effects:	Gastric erosion and bleeding, tinnitus, fever, thirst, diaphoresis
Dose:	325–650 mg PO q4–6h prn

IBUPROFEN (Advil, Motrin, Nuprin, and others)

Indications:	Pain due to inflammation, arthritis, soft tissue injury
Actions:	Interferes with production of prostaglandins
Side effects:	Nausea, diarrhea, gastric erosion and bleeding, dizziness, tinnitus
Dose:	400–800 mg PO tid to qid

INDOMETHACIN (Indocin, Indocin SR)

Indications:	Pain due to inflammation, arthritis, soft tissue injury, acute gout
Actions:	Interferes with production of prostaglandins
Side effects:	Gastric erosion and bleeding, dizziness, tinnitus, headache
Dose:	25 mg PO tid (Indocin); 75 mg PO bid (Indocin SR)

NAPROXEN (Naprosyn, Aleve)

Indications:	Pain due to inflammation, arthritis, soft tissue injury
Actions:	Interferes with production of prostaglandins
Side effects:	Nausea, diarrhea, gastric erosion and bleeding, dizziness, tinnitus
Dose:	250–500 mg bid

KETOROLAC (Toradol)

Indications:	Pain due to inflammation, arthritis, soft tissue injury
Actions:	Interferes with production of prostaglandins
Side effects:	Gastric erosion and bleeding, nausea, diarrhea, dizziness, tinnitus
Dose:	30–60 mg IM loading dose, followed by 15–30 mg IM q6h; maximum total daily dose is 120 mg, and the total recommended duration of therapy is 5 days; please note that the indication for oral ketorolac is only following prior IM administration.

APPENDIX B

ANTIBIOTIC STANDARD DOSES

Drug	Dosage Range (g/d) IV/IM*	Usual Dosage (grams per dosing interval) IV/IM*	Special Comments and Usage
Amikacin	15 mg/kg	7.5 mg/kg q12h	Good coverage for gram-negative rods Useful for organisms resistant to gentamicin and tobramycin Consider use in patients with gram-negative infections with contraindication to amino-glycoside use
Amoxicillin	1–6	0.5–1 q8h	Good for group B streptococcus, *Streptococcus viridans, Streptococcus pneumoniae,* and staphylococcus
Ampicillin	2–12	1 q6h	Drug of choice for enterococcus, group B streptococcus, *Listeria,* and actinomycete Useful for treatment of sepsis in combination with an aminoglycoside and either metronidazole or clindamycin

Table continued on following page

315

ANTIBIOTIC STANDARD DOSES *Continued*

Drug	Dosage Range (g/d) IV/IM*	Usual Dosage (grams per dosing interval) IV/IM*	Special Comments and Usage
Aztreonam	1–8	0.5–2 q8h	Good gram-negative coverage Consider use in patients with gram-negative infections with renal insufficiency or contraindication to aminoglycoside use
Cefazolin	3–6	1 q8h	Most common preoperative antibiotic Good *Staphylococcus aureus* and *Staphylococcus epidermis* coverage Moderate streptococcus groups A and B coverage Does not cover enterococcus
Cefotaxime	3–8	1–2 q6–8h	Moderate coverage of streptococcus and staphylococcus, but does not cover enterococcus Useful in meningitis because of gram-negative rods' resistance to ampicillin
Cefoxitin	3–6	1–2 q6–8h	Some staphylococcus and streptococcus coverage, and moderate anaerobic gram-positive (*Clostridium*) and anaerobic gram-negative coverage (*Bacteroides fragilis*) with a single agent
Ceftazidime	3–6	1 q8h	Good *Pseudomonas* coverage Consider use when gram-negative infection and aminoglycosides inappropriate
Ceftriaxone	1–4	1–2 q12–24h	Longer half-life than other cephalosporins Moderate staphylococcus and streptococcus coverage Useful in meningitis because of gram-negative rods' resistance to ampicillin
Cefuroxime	2–4.5	0.5–1 q8h	Mixed lung infections in penicillin-allergic patients *Haemophilus influenzae* resistant to ampicillin Good coverage for streptococcus and staphylococcus except MRSA and enterococcus

Drug	Dose*	Comments
Ciprofloxacin	0.4–0.8	200–400 mg q12h	Broad-spectrum agent for urinary tract infections and as adjunct for complicated skin infection; also, good bone penetration 500 mg PO q12h has bioavailability equal to 400 mg IV q12h
Clindamycin	0.6–2	0.6 q8h	Good coverage for anaerobes "above the diaphragm" *B. fragilis* dosing
Erythromycin	1–4	0.5 q6h	Drug of choice for *Legionella, Chlamydia, Mycoplasma* Moderate *S. aureus* and streptococcus groups A and B coverage Does not cover *S. epidermidis* or enterococcus
Gentamicin	3–5 mg/kg	1–1.5 mg/kg q8h	Serious aerobic gram-negative rod infections Follow gentamicin levels and creatinine
Imipenem	1–2	0.5 q6h	Good staphylococcus coverage, except MRSA Good anaerobic and aerobic enteric coverage Consider "big-gun agent"
Metronidazole	1–2	0.5 q8h	Good gram-negative enteric coverage Good for anaerobes "below the diaphragm" Well absorbed orally Good for pseudomembranous colitis caused by *Clostridium difficile*
Penicillin	2–20 mU	1–4 mU q4–6h	Drug of choice for streptococcal infections Good for oral infections, human bites, and anaerobic infections "above the diaphragm"
Piperacillin	6–12	1.5–2 q4h	*Pseudomonas* infections Moderate gram-negative enteric coverage
Tetracycline	1–2	0.5 q6h	Avoid use in children or pregnant patients because bone and tooth development are affected
Tobramycin	3–5 mg/kg	1.5 mg/kg q8h	More effective than gentamicin for *Pseudomonas* infection
Vancomycin	1–2	1 q12h	Drug of choice for MRSA Useful in multidrug-resistant gram-positive infections

*Unless otherwise specified.
MRSA = methicillin-resistant *Staphylococcus aureus*; mU = million units.
From Adams GA, Bresnick SD: On Call Surgery. Philadelphia, WB Saunders, 1997, pp 481–483.

INDEX

Note: Page numbers in *italics* refer to illustrations; page numbers followed by t refer to tables.